# Modern
# Caveman

## THE COMPLETE PALEO LIFESTYLE HANDBOOK

**BRETT L. MARKHAM**
the bestselling author of *Mini Farming*

Skyhorse Publishing

Skyhorse Publishing books may be purchased in bulk at special discounts for sales promotion, corporate gifts, fund-raising, or educational purposes. Special editions can also be created to specifications. For details, contact the Special Sales Department, Skyhorse Publishing, 307 West 36th Street, 11th Floor, New York, NY 10018 or info@ skyhorsepublishing.com.

Skyhorse® and Skyhorse Publishing® are registered trademarks of Skyhorse Publishing, Inc.®, a Delaware corporation.

Visit our website at www.skyhorsepublishing.com.

10 9 8 7 6 5 4 3 2 1

Library of Congress Cataloging-in-Publication Data is available on file.

ISBN: 978-1-62873-715-8

Printed in China

# Contents

Acknowledgments............................................................ v

Chapter 1: Why Question the Status Quo? ...................................... 1

Chapter 2: Fundamental Premises of the
Modern Caveman Diet................................... 13

Chapter 3: Why Legumes Should Come with
a Warning Label............................................. 27

Chapter 4: Why You Should Avoid Grains Like the Plague .............. 39

Chapter 5: Does Milk Do Your Body Good? ................................... 55

Chapter 6: Myths, Realities, and What You Need to
Know About Fats................................................ 75

Chapter 7: Carbohydrates: Dangerous Curves Ahead ..................... 101

Chapter 8: The Deadly White Powder ............................................. 115

Chapter 9: Meat's Back on the Menu ............................................. 135

Chapter 10: The Modern Caveman Food Pyramid.......................... 157

Chapter 11: Is It Caveman?............................................. 167

Chapter 12: Supermarket Checklists................................ 187

Chapter 13: Your Brain and Your Personal Environment................. 195

**Chapter 14:** Baseline Caveman Fitness .......................................... 209

**Chapter 15:** Caveman Flexibility ...................................................... 223

**Chapter 16:** Caveman Strength and Power ...................................... 245

**Chapter 17:** FAQs and Roadblocks ................................................. 285

**Index** .............................................................................................. 295

# Acknowledgments

This is no ordinary book. It tells you how to cure acne, improve your fertility, avoid premature wrinkles, take control of your genetic expression, keep your kids from ever getting multiple sclerosis, and stop most metastatic cancer. This book explains why practically everything most people take for granted about diet is not merely wrong but dangerously so.

When I was a kid, my father and paternal grandfather always made time to teach. They would discuss any topic I wanted, ranging from the nature of God to "what happens if you throw a baseball at 60 mph while standing on the front of a train traveling at the speed of light?" They taught me how to think critically and how to recognize my own implicit premises and subject them to critique.

This book questions everything from the wisdom of eating whole grains to the role of saturated fat and cholesterol in heart disease. It shows you that the very recommendations we get from doctors serve to make us sick. Without the influence of my father and grandfather, I can't be sure I'd have the confidence to write a book subjecting authority to such serious critique.

I need to thank my friend Adrianne Priest for planting the seeds that ultimately led not just to the ideas in this book but also to the full recovery of my health. My friend Lynn Pina kept telling me that I *had* to write this book because people needed it. My editor at Skyhorse Publishing, Jenn McCartney, convinced me to write this book sooner rather than later. My wife, Francine, did the editing and pointed out areas in which I was assuming common knowledge that wasn't common. My friend Rob Freeman contributed the Swiss ball stretches and continues to break new ground in the fields of balance, proprioception, and back health.

This is the first book for which I needed to take pictures of other people because it's hard for me to be on both sides of the lens at once. Consequently, I show up only in a few photographs. All of the other pictures are courtesy of three wonderful people.

I owe thanks (and a bottle of homemade wine) to my friend, coworker, and political debate partner Ruth Slater. Ruth is a fitness enthusiast who teaches rock climbing. She has an infectious smile and a positive attitude that really comes through in her back extensions. Thank you, Ruth!

Joel Bergeron graciously demonstrated a number of exercises. Joel is a fitness expert and real athlete with impressive credentials. It was a real joy to work with him because he understood exactly what I was trying to demonstrate, the proper form and the proper angles. The photo of kettlebell swings was taken with him holding the kettlebell straight out in front, still in proper form, so the picture wouldn't be blurred. This takes a lot of strength. Thank you, Joel!

Just before this book was due, I discovered I was missing some pictures I needed. Chaunty Spillane is a model, actress, and yoga enthusiast. Her experience with yoga was perfect because she already knew every exercise I needed her to demonstrate, and she did it perfectly the first time. She held the flying pose with perfect balance while I properly framed the shot. Chaunty was great to work with and brought a lot of fun to the track. Thank you, Chaunty!

# Chapter 1
# Why Question the Status Quo?

William Dampier, Walter Raleigh, Abel Tasman, and James Cook are not exactly household names today, but they were explorers who chronicled their experiences in meeting people from hunter-gatherer cultures. One thing that stands out in their writings is that they uniformly described the hunter-gatherers they encountered all over the world as being healthy, strong, and well muscled.

In his *A New Voyage Round the World*, Dampier describes the Moskito people he encountered in the following manner: "They are tall, well made, raw-boned, lusty, strong, and nimble of foot." Abel Tasman's description of the Maori people of New Zealand gives one the impression of Olympic gymnasts or high-level mixed martial arts fighters. Joseph Bank's description of Australians encountered on James Cook's journey notes that "they were of a common size, lean and seemed active and nimble."

This is hardly a fluke. Prior to the dawn of agriculture, humans had brains 20 percent larger on average than we do today.[1] Considering that hunter-gatherers were the original inventors who laid the groundwork for language and art that we have inherited, it might not be surprising they had larger brains.

Though there are a number of theories for our decreased cranial capacity, and scientists like everyone else are often constrained to protect people's feelings, the predominant theory is that the grain-based civilization enabled larger population densities and a specialized world in which average people didn't have to be as smart to survive.[2] Even among modern populations,

---

[1] J. Hawkes, *Selection for Smaller Brains in Holocene Human Evolution*

[2] D. Bailey and D. Geary, "Hominid Brain Evolution: Testing Climatic, Ecological and Social Competition Models," *Human Nature* 20 (2009): 67–79.

the negative nutritional impact on the brain of excluding meat from the diet in favor of grains and legumes can be seen quite starkly.[3]

Because this point is debated, it might not be enough to convince you. So let me ask: When was the last time you visited the dentist, and how much did it cost? From fossil studies, it has been consistently demonstrated that our preagricultural forebears had a virtual absence of tooth decay.[4] Scientists analyzing skeletons from Sudan determined that the percentage of the population afflicted with tooth decay was less than 1 percent as hunter-gatherers, but the predominance of dental caries skyrocketed to 20 percent of the population upon the adoption of grain-based agriculture.[5] Cavities are something we accept as a fact of life today, but given a diet that matches our evolutionary character, they either do not occur or are healed as they happen. Yes, given an ancestral diet, our bodies can actually heal cavities.[6, 7]

One very common objection to caveman diets is that the diets were fine for cavemen in the short run because cavemen only lived to be twenty-five to thirty-five years old. This line of reasoning reveals a misunderstanding of both statistics and causality. In hunter-gatherer cultures without access to medical care, child mortality is very high, with about half of children dying before age fifteen. This is what you'd expect in a relatively primitive environment without access to vaccines or modern medicine. How many of our children (and mothers) would have died except for modern

---

[3] A. Vogiatzoglou et al., "Vitamin B12 Status and Rate of Brain Volume Loss in Community-Dwelling Elderly," *Neurology* 71, no. 11 (2008): 826–32.

[4] K. Gruber, "Oral Mystery: Are Agriculture and Rats Responsible for Tooth Decay?" *Scientific American*, February 6, 2013.

[5] D. L. Greene G. H. Ewing, and G. J. Armelagos, "Dentition of a Mesolithic Population from Wadi Halfa, Sudan." *American Journal of Physical Anthropology* 27 (1967): 41–55.

[6] W. Price, *Nutrition and Physical Degeneration* (La Mesa, CA: Price-Pottenger Nutrition, 2008).

[7] R. Nagel, *Cure Tooth Decay: Heal And Prevent Cavities With Nutrition— Limit and Avoid Dental Surgery and Fluoride*, 2d ed. (Ashland, OR: Golden Child Publishing, 2010).

surgery and the Caesarian section? How many of our children would have perished from whooping cough, tetanus, or smallpox without vaccines? How many of our children would have died from ear infections or infections from a compound fracture were it not for modern antibiotics? Yes, the *average* lifespan of a caveman was twenty-five to thirty-five years but only because of infant and child mortality in primitive medical conditions.

But as hunter-gatherers get older and successfully avoid myriad hazards, their life expectancy increases to about age seventy-two.[8] Though this isn't exactly ancient by modern standards, it's also a lot older than stereotypes would lead us to believe and plenty old enough to indicate that their diet didn't kill them off by age thirty-five. This is especially true given their lack of access to medical care. If you take away antibiotics, life-saving surgeries following accidents, vaccinations, antivenin for snakebites, and similar innovations, it's doubtful our average lifespan would be very long either.

In fact, the results of a comprehensive archeological symposium on the health of Paleolithic and Mesolithic humans concluded, "Taken as a whole, these indicators fairly clearly suggest an overall decline in the quality—and probably in the length—of human life associated with the adoption of agriculture."[9]

The aforementioned archaeological symposium took place in the 1980s, long before anyone put forward the idea of paleo, ancestral, or caveman diets or seriously considered that a hunter-gatherer diet might be ideal for our nutritional needs, yet the book compiled from that symposium sounds like an advertisement for such diets. For example:

In Upper Paleolithic times nutritional health was excellent. The evidence consists of extremely tall stature from plentiful

---

[8] M. Gurven and H. Kaplan, "Longevity Among Hunter-Gatherers: A Cross-Cultural Examination, Population and Development," *Review* 33, no. 2 (2007): 321–65.

[9] M. N. Cohen MN and G. J. Armelagos, *Paleopathology and the Origins of Agriculture* (London: Academic Press, 1984).

calories and protein; maximum skull base height from plentiful protein, vitamin D, and sunlight in early childhood; and very good teeth and large pelvic depth from adequate protein and vitamins in later childhood and adolescence. . . . There is no clear evidence for any endemic disease.[10]

In another part of the book, the researchers point out that the switch from a hunter-gatherer diet sacrificed the nutritional value of the individual in order to support a higher population density.

Early nonagricultural diets appear to have been high in minerals, protein, vitamins, and trace nutrients, but relatively low in starch. In the development toward agriculture there is a growing emphasis on starchy, highly caloric food of high productivity and storability, changes that are not favorable to nutritional quality but that would have acted to increase carrying capacity.

This, then, is the key to understanding the current dominant diet recommendations supported by governments. These recommendations focus on caloric sources such as grains that can be produced abundantly and cheaply, supporting a higher number of human beings at lower cost. But these are the same caloric sources used to fatten up feedlot cattle for slaughter, representing a preference for quantity over quality. Obviously, the higher population density of humans that agriculture enabled came with benefits in terms of leisure, specialization, and technological progress. I am not advocating a return to the primitive. Rather, my aim is much smaller: to persuade *you* that your *individual* health would benefit from adopting a modern caveman diet.

## My Saga

Toward that end, I am going to explain the personal saga that got me interested in ancestral diets in the first place. Along the

---

[10] Ibid.

way, I will explain what led me to question the status quo and why you should question it too.

At the ripe old age of thirty-six, my primary care doctor informed me that I had borderline high blood pressure and if I didn't get my cholesterol under control, I'd be dead in short order. My inflammation markers were sky-high as well. The thing is, I had been eating what might have been the world's most politically correct diet. I was already eating a diet that was supposed to keep my cholesterol down.

I was eating tofurkey. I was eating lots of whole grains. In fact, I would literally take whole wheat kernels and cook them mixed with ("heart healthy") oatmeal in a thermos overnight. I eschewed all forms of animal fat and only ate "healthy" fats like canola oil. I drank soy milk and rice milk. I would make pot after pot of beans rather than eat the meat I had been told would kill me. I combined it with corn bread to make a "complete protein." I was very close to being a vegetarian.

When I explained this to my doctor, he shrugged and said I was doing all the right things but simply had "bad genes" and would need to go on statin drugs right away and stay on them for the rest of my life.

What's worse, even though my doctor's reasoning was incorrect, I could feel in my own body that I was heading nowhere fast. Even though I had been an accomplished martial artist (and was still actively involved in martial arts), had run hurdles in high school and college, and had generally maintained what everyone says is an ideal lifestyle, I was in pain every day.

My joints hurt, particularly my knees. The bottoms of my feet were so tender that I would wince when I stepped. I had nearly constant gastrointestinal pain that would often debilitate me for days. I kept trying to eat vegetables, but my gastrointestinal tract couldn't hack most of them, so I took vitamins.

I had no doubt that my doctor was right about my eminent demise, but I was unconvinced about the need for statins and doubly convinced that there was nothing wrong with my genes. One thing I knew was that Mother Nature didn't invest millions of years in my evolution so my genome would be incompatible with a healthy lifestyle.

So I started digging. My doctor had told me that my "bad genes" were going to kill me in spite of eating a diet that would make the American Heart Association proud, and his solution to the problem was to give me drugs that would compensate for my "bad genes." It never even occurred to him to question *the diet*. When I looked up the potential side effects of the statin drugs my doctor wanted to prescribe, they included memory loss, impotence, muscle pain, and more. It seemed to me that medication of that sort should be an absolute last resort because it had the potential to make my life barely worth living at an early age.

Remembering my experience with lactose and the food pyramid (I am lactose intolerant, so it is absurd for the government to specify that I need milk to be healthy), and having read a couple of philosophy books in my life, I considered that it might be time to *question my premises*. That is, it was time to question the premise that the food recommendations put forward by the USDA and my doctor were optimal for my genes rather than question the quality of my genes.

Thus, I embarked on a mission to understand what was wrong with my diet. Though my home lab would impress a kid, it wouldn't impress a scientist at a modern university, because the technology is largely 1950s and homemade. Instead of a gas chromatograph and mass spectrometer, I use thin-layer chromatography and a homemade light spectrometer that uses a prism from an old periscope. I used microcontrollers, heating elements, and an old cooler to make my own incubator. My microbiological techniques were straight out of the 1940s and 1950s. Still, I set out on my quest with the gear I could build myself and a desire to figure out what was wrong.

Because I had so many intestinal problems and was often in pain from them, I figured that would be a good place to start. I remembered reading an old medical book from the 1800s in which doctors described a phenomenon known to them as "autointoxication," in which ordinary gut bacteria went awry and made people sick. Doctors did a lot of "purging" back in those days—usually with nasty stuff nobody should ever consume—but purging was the treatment, so I tested the results of taking saline laxatives, and sure enough, fasting and then purging with a laxative made me feel better until shortly after I started eating again.

I realized that, political correctness aside, something was wrong with what I was eating. I won't bore you with the endless details of my experiments in a primitive laboratory and will instead cut to the chase of the personal saga. Within a few years, I had made headway and was doing somewhat better by eliminating soy and wheat from my diet, but it took one more step for me to make the leap into ancestral diet.

Though I had made some progress in researching diet on my own the hard way, a few years ago my friend Adrianne asked my opinion on the theories of a veterinarian who calls himself Dogtor J. Though my research had produced a number of valuable conclusions—including the finding that I shouldn't be eating soy or wheat—those conclusions weren't linked by a cohesive principle that would allow me to extrapolate and generalize, because I was mired in germ theory (the interactions between food, gut bacteria, the compounds they produce, and the effects on health) and had insufficient resources to move forward. Dogtor J provided the unifying insight linking my discoveries together into something that made sense: evolution.

Dogtor J's ideas are the same fundamentals that underlie caveman diet: Evolution isn't a fast process, so we are genetically optimized for the diet consumed by our distant hunter-gatherer forebears. Depending on which authority is consulted, the human family tree separated from other primates about four and a half million years ago, whereas modern agricultural staples entered our diet only six thousand years ago or even less in many cases.

As a result, our predominant genes are more compatible with the diet of hunter-gatherers than with the heavily grain-based diets we currently consume. In other words, *instead of faulting our genes for being incompatible with the diet we feed cattle in order to fatten them up for slaughter, we should adapt our diet to meet the needs of the genes we already have.*

How is my health? Eleven years have passed since my doctor's dire prediction. I am taking no regular medications. I have only rarely been ill at all. I no longer have constant pain, my digestion works great, and I feel better than I did when I was thirty. My blood pressure is what it was when I entered a military academy at age eighteen.

*My life has been transformed, and I believe what is contained in this book can transform your life as well.*

## Question Everything

The man who was my doctor when I was thirty-six is a good man. He's a man of science, absolutely brilliant, and undoubtedly well-intentioned. If I were to die, I wouldn't mind having him raise my child in my stead. How is it that he gave me such bad advice?

As a student of science, I have read hundreds of books on the sciences—including books that are hundreds of years old. One thing that stands out is that at each stage of our development, we considered ourselves to be at the pinnacle of human knowledge while ridiculing the knowledge accepted only a few decades prior.

This is evident in those sciences pertaining to human health. It is interesting to read a medical book from the 1920s excoriate prior practitioners for using leeches while simultaneously advocating the use of arsenic to treat infections. Those doctors had no idea that today we would look with horror upon the mercury and arsenic they used routinely. Most people of science today act without realization that one hundred years from now, it is likely that much of what they believe so steadfastly today will also have been proven wrong.

Another thing that stands out, oddly enough, is an amazing degree of conformity with the accepted ideas of the day. Sometimes progress in the most basic of matters takes decades. One instance that comes to mind is ulcers. A doctor in the 1950s demonstrated quite clearly that stomach ulcers were caused by a bacterium and could be cured with antibiotics. Because he stood outside the mainstream beliefs of his day, he was ignored, and ulcers were treated surgically (and many people suffered and died needlessly) for many decades thereafter until—of all things—an article in the *National Enquirer* called attention to the pointless costs and deaths of this modality.[11]

Conformity in sciences is the rule rather than the exception. Conformity is not always bad, because it allows us to have a society in which we are confident in our ability to be physically safe. For example, almost everyone agrees that attacking other people is wrong. Without broad conformity on this issue, it is doubtful human societies could even exist. Even so, enforced conformity has likely been a major cause of delays in the advancement of human knowledge in nearly every field, and these delays harm people who could benefit from improved knowledge. No field makes this more obvious today than the field of diet.

In 2012, Dr. John Ioannidis of Stanford University and Joshua Nicholson of Virginia Tech published a paper entitled "Research Grants: Conform and Be Funded."[12] Though human limitations mean any analysis of practically anything will be less than perfect, the authors demonstrated that in the life sciences, the most influential, innovative, and cited research was the *least* likely to be funded and that funding tended to enforce conformity with existing views.

The unfortunate truth of their contention can be demonstrated by the fact that our medical, scientific, and lay communities uncritically accept a number of premises regarding health that are far from absolutely true and often outright false. In fact, if you have previously accepted the current standard views on diet and health, you will soon read convincing evidence that much of what you have been told is wrong.

---

[11] P. Ewald, *The New Germ Theory of Disease* (New York: Anchor Books, 2002).

[12] J. Ionnidis and J. Nicholson, "Research Grants: Conform and Be Funded," *Nature* 492 (2012): 34–36.

Obviously, it is not practical for each of us to individually confirm every belief that we hold. Not only would it be inordinately time consuming but it's also not realistic to expect that we all have the tools, equipment, training, and funding to double-check things. So we rely on experts. The problem is that the experts also rely on experts. The end results were my being in constant pain and my doctor recommending the very things that had put me in that condition in the first place—and the recommendation to take medication that had the potential to destroy the quality of my life as a solution.

## Why I Wrote This Book

After exploring Dogtor J's ideas, I started finding some books on Paleolithic or caveman diet. The books were very valuable in describing in detail the reasons why we shouldn't be eating grain, but these books also had frustrating deficiencies. For example, though the books posited that we ought not eat legumes, they tended to focus their reasoning for that proscription on soy alone and ignored detailing why we shouldn't eat other legumes.

But perhaps the largest deficiency lay in the fact that although the authors at least had the fortitude to effectively question an entire scientific establishment on the wisdom of eating grains, legumes, and dairy, they uncritically accepted the established party lines on saturated fat, cholesterol, and salt among other things. They ignored or barely addressed the role of diet in mental health and completely ignored the role of gut microbes in health. They failed to distinguish between omega-3s from plants and omega-3s from animals—and that distinction is crucial. In some cases, their dietary lists even excluded foods that cause no problems and have been shown to be healthy. In other cases, the guidelines specified foods that were too expensive for most people to afford—particularly for a family. Most of the books also ignored the flip side of diet: exercise.

So, that was why I wrote this book. The underlying evolutionary principles of a caveman diet are entirely valid, but we do not live in

Paleolithic times; the recommendations have to be consonant with what is practical and affordable for people. Furthermore, existing works in my opinion are sound to the extent that they question established dietary guidelines, but they *do not go far enough in their questioning.*

Nature is an amazing artisan. You were designed to be healthy, strong, and happy. You are already halfway there because you have nature's amazing design in the DNA contained within the cells of your body. All you have to do is give that DNA the materials and conditions it was optimized to use, and you'll see the results.

Finally, I have a disclaimer before we dive into the meat of things. This book represents my opinions based on research. I am not a medical doctor and nothing in this book is intended to diagnose or treat any disease. Parts of this book discuss exercise. You should get a physical exam and clearance from your doctor before undertaking any exercise program.

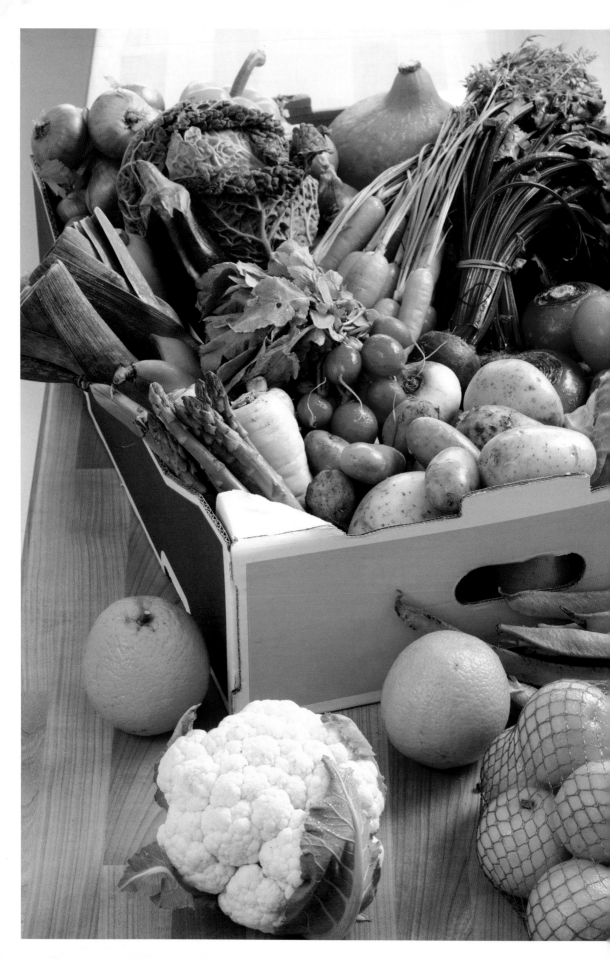

# Chapter 2
# Fundamental Premises of the Modern Caveman Diet

## Evolution, Groups, and Individuals

The fundamental premise of the caveman diet is as simple as evolution. In fact, it *is* evolution. Human beings separated from other primates somewhere in the neighborhood of four million years ago. Over those four million years, we coevolved with a hunter-gatherer diet. Over the past 6,000 to 10,000 years, we have developed large-scale agriculture that has shifted our dietary intake from that of hunter-gatherers to that of an agricultural and herding society. The idea behind the caveman diet is that evolution is not a particularly fast process and that, in general, our bodies are better adapted to thrive on what we consumed for 98 percent of our specifically human evolution as opposed to what we have consumed for the latter 2 percent of our evolution.

Every other idea in the caveman diet is a corollary of this evolutionary premise. In general, caveman diet supposes that the predominant foods of civilization combined with our current sedentary lifestyle gives rise to the so-called diseases of civilization, such as metabolic disorder.

The premises of a caveman diet are imperfect. For example, early humans occupied a variety of ecological niches. One group of humans may have eaten more seafood, whereas another would have eaten more herbivores. Humans closer to the equator would have had more access to fruit, whereas humans closer to the Arctic would have had little access. As a result, there would be differences in adaptation.

These differences in adaptation can be seen in individual differences in food tolerance to this very day. Because of this, it is impossible for me to say with extreme specificity that you, in particular, should eat lobster. For all I know, you may have a shellfish allergy that would make eating lobster your last fatal mistake. Therefore, while there are matters I can and will address broadly, it is more important that you pay attention to the principles rather than the specifics.

A related imperfection in the caveman diet is that it fails to account for individual differences in genetics. Though evolution is slow, it *can* respond swiftly in the face of selection pressures. You can see this in our selective breeding of everything from chickens to crops. If you feed people a diet containing something harmful, over time those who survive will be better adapted to the new diet than those who died. This is no different from the phenomenon of antibiotic resistance. A given antibiotic may kill nearly all bacteria of a certain variety, but those that survive will ultimately give rise to descendants who aren't harmed by that antibiotic at all. This level of adaptation does not, however, render the historical diet harmful; it just makes the new diet less than immediately lethal.

One example of this is the ability to digest lactose. Though most humans worldwide can't digest lactose by the time they reach adulthood, there are segments of humanity who digest lactose with sufficient ease to keep ice cream manufacturers in business. In fact, individuals from the various segments of humanity who have the ability to digest lactose have gained that ability through distinctly different genetic pathways,[1] demonstrating convergent evolution within a relatively short time span of 6,000 to 10,000 years.

This indicates that, to some degree anyway, human evolution has adapted to cope with the foodstuffs of the agricultural and herding diet that followed our caveman diet. This means that though the caveman diet has a scientific basis that is as sound as evolution, there will be aspects that will differ as a result of more recent evolutionary pressures affecting humanity in different locales.

Every human is a unique individual and a product of a slightly different genetic path than any other person on earth.

---

[1] S. A. Tishkoff *et al.*, "Convergent Adaptation of Human Lactase Persistence in Africa and Europe," *Nature Genetics* 39, no. 1 (2007): 31–40.

Though some broad correlations can be drawn between certain dietary adaptations and population groups, such correlations are irrelevant on an individual basis because nobody completely conforms to any given average. As but one example, my ancestry is wholly European and about half of that is from Ireland and Britain. Based on this, you'd assume I can digest lactose, but, in fact, I cannot. So the degree and details of post-Paleolithic adaptations are very individual and can't be easily ascertained simply on the basis of superficial factors.

Blood type diets also fall short. Though they attempt to compensate for differences in individual genetics, the science behind them is scanty at best, and the fundamental premises are flawed. For example, the blood type diet assumes that blood type O is the oldest human blood type, whereas microbiological analysis indicates that type A is likely the oldest.[2] There is no correlation between dietary adaptations for which we can test and a person's blood type except in a fashion that is so broad as to be useless to an individual.

So a common failure of approaches to the caveman diet is that they assume all humans are identical, that all of their evolution stopped 10,000 years ago, and that thus they should all eat the same things. Though this is certainly broadly applicable, when you get down to details, every person is a bit different. Even so, the primary premise of the caveman diet is that even though there has been *some* evolution since caveman times, the degree of evolution has not been so great as to negate the benefits of eating as our ancestors did.

## The Core Caveman Diet

When people ask me to explain the caveman diet, they are shocked that the explanation is so simple. You can eat meat, fish,

---

[2] N. Saitou and F. Yamamoto, "Evolution of Primate ABO Blood Group Genes and Their Homologous Genes," *Molecular Biology and Evolution* 14, no. 4 (1997): 399–411

eggs, fruits, nuts, and vegetables. In other words, you can eat everything that a hunter-gatherer in the Paleolithic era could have eaten. You can't eat grains, legumes, most dairy, or anything that requires the artifacts of Neolithic or later civilizations to produce. This latter category includes refined sugars, most (though not all) vegetable oils, and chemicals whose names most people would have difficulty pronouncing. Should you eat FD & C Blue #1? Can you roll its chemical name off your tongue? Ethyl-[4-[[4-[ethyl-[(3-sulfophenyl)methyl]amino]phenyl]-(2-sulfophenyl)methylidene]-1-cyclohexa-2,5-dienylidene]-[(3-sulfophenyl)methyl]azanium. No? Me neither. So we shouldn't eat it. It's that simple.

In theory, the previous paragraph is all you need to know. With just that information, you can follow a caveman diet and derive its myriad benefits. If a substance is questionable, you merely need to ask if it could have been produced in a hunter-gatherer tribe 20,000 years ago.

For example, should you eat tapioca? Tapioca comes from the manioc root. If you eat the tuber raw, you will die from cyanide poisoning. In order to be made edible, manioc root is processed extensively in a fashion that would have been impossible in a preagricultural society. Hence, it is not allowed. Of course, there are other reasons you shouldn't eat tapioca, the most notable of which is that it is a nutritionally vapid pure carbohydrate that will raise your blood sugar, trigger an insulin response, and—unless you are eating it immediately following vigorous physical activity such that your muscles are depleted of glycogen—it will turn into fat in your body in short order.

At the same time, though the logic of Paleolithic eating works for a great many things, it could do you a disservice if applied religiously. For example, should you use vinegar as a condiment? Since making vinegar in useful quantities would have required a fixed-location lifestyle unachievable before the dawn of agriculture, a strict interpretation would exclude it from your diet. But is there any reason to exclude it beyond that? No. In fact, there is substantial evidence that vinegar in moderation is a beneficial addition to your diet.

And that is why this book is called *Modern Caveman*. The ideas underlying the caveman diet are applied, but they are applied in light of modern knowledge. Because of this, instead of the two categories of "Eat" and "Don't Eat," there is also a third category called "Eat in Moderation" as well as a fourth category called "Eat with Caution."

## Caveman Moderation

In an age when superlatives are employed so ubiquitously that saying something is "good" rather than "super fantastic" runs the risk of being an insult, I find that the concept of moderation doesn't have a good anchor for understanding. What, exactly, is moderation as it pertains to a modern caveman diet?

Honey is something to which cavemen likely had access. They didn't keep their own hives, of course. But if they encountered a wild hive and were willing to brave thousands of stings, they could have had some honey. And because honey is naturally preserved, they could have taken it home and shared it with their tribe. But in practice, you'd have to ask yourself, how often could a hive be found and readily accessible? Once a hive was discovered, how many cavemen would willingly endure the life-threatening risk of thousands of stings in order to acquire it? Though stingless bees exist, their honey is of inferior keeping quality, so how widely could such honey have been shared?

Likewise, vinegar was encountered in the natural world. If you have ever been under an apple tree in the fall, you have undoubtedly noticed the distinct smell of vinegar in the air from fallen and partially rotted fruit. Putting yourself in a caveman's bare feet, how likely would you be to eat that fruit? Under what circumstances would you eat it? Some perfectly fine fruit could have been brought back to the cave and stockpiled for winter before it subsequently started to rot.

It should be obvious that moderation does not mean something you eat by the bucket loads every day.

Practically all diets provide some benefits to their adherents. The reason is that following nearly any set diet at least introduces consciousness of what we put in our mouths and a degree of *intention* and *planning*. Nearly any rational diet tells you that broccoli is a better nutritional choice than ice cream. The reason most diets are very strict is because if something is "allowed with moderation," it quickly becomes a mainstay of the diet and sabotages the benefits of consciousness and intentionality.

I recently read a study of Seventh Day Adventists indicating that those who followed a vegetarian diet had a 12 percent reduced risk of death.[3] Obviously, eating nothing but pure sugar day in and day out would constitute being a vegetarian, and it should be equally obvious that such a diet would be unhealthy. The key to the modest comparative benefit of Seventh Day Adventist vegetarians over more or less random eaters is given in the article when it says that the religion "promotes somewhat strict dietary rules"—in other words, intentionality. As I said, practically any consciously adopted and intentional diet with rules and guidelines will be superior to the willy-nilly "eat whatever tastes good" approach that the population as a whole takes to eating.

So it becomes important for me to define moderation in a fashion that won't allow it to subvert the overall diet.

In general, in the United States, people eat three meals a day, or twenty-one meals a week. During *three* of the twenty-one meals, you can eat one or more things that are allowed "in moderation." The other eighteen meals cannot include such items.

Why did I pick three instead of two or four? There is no scientifically supportable reason. It's just that human nature requires limits, and I chose that limit because it balances between the benefits of strict dietary adherence, the desire for dietary variety, and the pitfalls of prohibition.

## Caveman Caution

Caution is warranted anytime you deal with a foodstuff that would have been unavailable in useful quantities or with regularity in a hunter-gatherer society.

There are a couple of reasons why caution is warranted.

---

[3] A. Singh, "Could That Steak Be Killing You? Vegetarianism Proven to Increase Life Expectancy," *Medical Daily*, June 3, 2013.

The first reason is that, though humans have clearly made *some* adaptations in the past 10,000 years, those adaptations are by no means comprehensive, complete, or universal. Hence, the foods may not be compatible with health simply due to our lack of adaptation.

The near-universal recommendations for yogurt consumption as a means of replenishing healthy gut flora fall along those lines. Not only does most yogurt contain only one or two live bacterial strains (out of a potential of thousands) but also most popular yogurt brands contain an astonishing 4.3 grams of pure sugar per ounce. As a point of comparison, Coca Cola contains 3.25 grams of sugar per ounce, or 25 percent less than the sweetened yogurt[4] people usually buy. Even worse, unlike aged cheeses, yogurt contains enough lactose that it can't be digested by lactose-intolerant people. How did people replenish their gut flora back before containers of sealed yogurt became available?

Another example would be shellfish. Some human populations developed near shellfish and others didn't. As a result, some people can't safely eat shellfish.

The second reason is that more modern food creations are vastly different from our ancestral diet in important ways. For example, the wild game that formed a core of our ancestral diet has a much more favorable ratio of omega-6 to omega-3 fatty acids than most of the meat sold today in the supermarket. Likewise, products such as canola oil may seem healthy, but once you understand that whatever omega-3 fats were there in the beginning have been rendered useless through processing at over 500 degrees in order to deodorize the product and make it palatable, it becomes apparent that such a product should be used with caution if at all.

## Evolutionary Self-Protection

Another idea underlying the caveman diet is that of evolutionary self-protection. Animals have self-protective attributes to avoid

---

[4] Data obtained from the Yoplait and Coca Cola websites comparing original Yoplait yogurt with original Coke.

being eaten. Whether it is the natural camouflage of a fawn, the poison of a rattlesnake, the smell of a skunk, or the speed of a cheetah, the defenses of animals are both obvious and well understood.

What is less obvious in many cases is that plants have also developed an impressive array of defenses to assure the survival of offspring.

Some plants, such as water hemlock, are outright poisonous, and no part of them can be eaten. Many other plants bear fruit that is delicious and edible, but their seeds contain poisons. (This way the fruit is eaten, and when the seed is discarded, the plant is propagating itself.) Examples of edible fruits with poisonous seeds include apples, peaches, and cherries. In some cases the seeds may be wholesome and appealing but coevolved with forgetful hoarders, such as squirrels, that spread the seeds by burying caches that are forgotten.

Seeds tend to be the most problematic part of plants as that is where plants tend to concentrate the protection of their offspring. In some cases, the protection is very obvious, as with the bristling spines surrounding a chestnut. In other cases, the protection is insidious, such as the hormonal disruptors in soybeans that inhibit the fertility of whatever is eating them.

The important idea is that the protection might be very obvious, such as spikes and spines, somewhat less obvious, as in a quick and deadly poison, or it could be hidden, such as the presence of antinutrients or hormonal disruptors that act subtly and aren't particularly obvious.

In other cases, the seeds are coated with substances that stop digestive enzymes so that when consumed by birds or other animals, they are excreted intact. If you have ever seen bird feces on your car, especially of the purple variety, you may have noticed a large number of small but intact seeds embedded in the material. Those seeds have a coating that makes them impervious to digestion. If you were to eat a large quantity of them with other foods, your digestion in general would be disrupted, you'd get a case of diarrhea, and you'd excrete those seeds along with some nice fertilizer.

But what if you were to chew the seeds thoroughly, grind them into a fine powder, or otherwise render the protective coating of the seed inoperative? On the positive side, your body would have an opportunity to absorb the internal content of the seed, including proteins and minerals. On the negative side, the seed materials that made it indigestible would be released to inhibit digestion generally, and any dangerous things in the seed would be accessible to absorption as well.

Obviously, it depends on the seed. If you were to swallow a castor bean whole, in most cases its digestion inhibitors would lead you to pass it in your stool intact, and you'd be okay. But if you were to grind it into a fine powder and eat it, you would die because of the poison[5] it contains. On the other hand, if you were to chew up the seeds in a grape you were eating, you'd absorb the beneficial phenolic compound resveratrol.

Grains and legumes are seeds. I'll be dedicating individual chapters on why you shouldn't eat them, but for now it should be understood that nature didn't leave grains and legumes defenseless and that unlike humanity's partial adaptation to dairy products, our adaptations to grains and legumes are insufficient for them to be consumed without causing harm.

Though the risks posed by beans are myriad, one of the more obvious risks is that nearly all beans contain a lectin called phytohaemagglutinin that poses a risk of acute poisoning unless it is deactivated.

As with beans, the defenses of grains are diverse, but one of the more immediate problems is that grains are high in phytic acid. Though many plants contain phytic acid, grains are particularly problematic in that regard because they contain few compensatory nutrients and are usually eaten in large quantities. Phytic acid stymies protein digestion by deactivating pepsin in the stomach[6]

---

[5] The poison in castor beans is a lectin called ricin. It is deadly, and in many cases even the best medical care cannot help.

[6] S. R. Tannenbaum, V. R. Young, and M. C. Archer, "Vitamins and Minerals, in Food Chemistry," in *Food Chemistry*, ed. O. R. Fennema, 2d ed. (New York: Marcel Dekker, 1985), 445.

and trypsin in the small intestine[7] while binding to important minerals so they can't be absorbed. Though the harm from this isn't so immediate as to be obvious, the long-term effects are not healthful.

Ruminant animals such as cows, incidentally, have gut bacteria that create phytase, which deactivates the phytic acid so they can eat grains without those long-term effects. Cows and humans simply evolved differently, and so what is good for one is not necessarily good for the other.

The key idea, then, is that a modern caveman diet takes into account the evolved defenses of plants and the degree to which human evolution has allowed us to compensate for those defenses. In cases in which our compensatory abilities are inadequately developed, the food is unhealthful and should be excluded other than to avoid immediate risks of starvation.

## A General Look at Lectins

Lectins are proteins that very specifically bind to particular types of sugar molecules. They are present in all plants and animals (including humans) and are used for a variety of internal processes. It would be impossible to eat without consuming lectins, and most of them are harmless to humans. From a food perspective, they are most common in grains, legumes, nuts, and potatoes. Those in nuts and potatoes are harmless to those who aren't sensitive to them, but the lectins in legumes and grains can be quite harmful both immediately and on a long-term basis.

The immediate harm from lectins is sufficiently obvious, and wise people avoid substances that contain them. Examples range from lectins in uncooked beans that result in nonfatal vomiting to the lectin solanine in green potatoes that can cause poisoning.

The long-term adverse effects of less obviously dangerous lectins are subtler. Lectins can be absorbed intact directly into

---

[7] M. Singh and D. Krikorian, "Inhibition of Trypsin Activity In Vitro by Phytate," *Journal of Agricultural and Food Chemistry* 30, no. 4 (1982): 799–800.

the bloodstream from the intestinal tract, including the lectins of legumes such as peanuts.[8] Most proteins that we consume are broken down by digestive enzymes into their constituent amino acids before being absorbed into the bloodstream from the small intestine. So in an ideal world, lectins could never be absorbed through the intestinal wall.

But the lectins in beans and grains can be absorbed into your body without being broken down. There are a number of reasons for this. First, beans and grains are high in phytic acid. Phytic acid is present to some degree in nearly all plants, but beans and grains contain very high concentrations of phytic acid and, in addition, tend to be consumed in large quantities. The high phytic acid concentrations stop the activity of the digestive enzymes that break down proteins, thus leaving the lectins in beans and grains intact.

Second, the lectins strip away the protective layer of mucus that lines the intestinal tract.[9] Not only does this phenomenon have adverse implications in terms of promoting growth of unfriendly bacteria that cause ulcers and other problems but it also allows substances to be absorbed that would otherwise be trapped in the mucus layer.

Finally, lectins—and this is their most insidious characteristic— often superficially resemble proteins native to the body. This means they are allowed into the bloodstream before their foreign nature is recognized.

Why should you care if lectins are absorbed into your bloodstream rather than being broken down to their constituent amino acids while within the intestines? Because their superficial resemblance to your native proteins that gets them past the guards and into your bloodstream in the first place means that when they are finally recognized as foreign invaders, your immune defenses might also attack the tissues in your body that the lectins resemble. This results in autoimmune diseases of various sorts.

---

[8] Q. Wang *et al.*, "Identification of Intact Peanut Lectin in Peripheral Venous Blood, *Lancet* 352 (1998): 1831–32.

[9] J. G. Banwell *et al.*, "Bacterial Overgrowth by Indigenous Microflora in the PHA-Fed Rat," *Canadian Journal of Microbiology* 34 (1988): 1009–13.

Examples of autoimmune diseases in which lectins are a risk factor include IgA nephropathy,[10] rheumatoid arthritis,[11, 12, 13, 14] and insulin-dependent diabetes.[15]

Because everyone is slightly genetically different and therefore might not be vulnerable to a specific lectin, it cannot be predicted with certainty that X lectin from Y food will cause Z illness in Ms. Jane Doe #53. What I can say is that, in general, grains and legumes contain lectins that pose an increased risk of autoimmune disorders, and you consume them at your peril. Two researchers stated the matter plainly:

> Of the food lectins, grain/cereal lectins, dairy lectins, and legume lectins are the most common ones associated with aggravation of inflammatory and digestive diseases in the body and improvement of these diseases and/or symptoms when avoided. Recent research has suggested that these lectins may effectively serve as a vehicle allowing foreign proteins to invade our natural gut defenses and cause damage well beyond the gut, commonly in joints, brain, skin, and various body glands. With continued exposure of the gut by these toxic food lectins a persistent stimulation of the body's

---

[10] R. Coppo, A. Amore, and D. Roccatello, "Dietary Antigens and Primary IgA Nephropathy," *Journal of the American Society of Nephrology* 2, suppl. 10 (1992): S173–S180.

[11] A. Bond, M. A. Kerr, and F. C. Hay, "Distinct Oligosaccharide Content of Rheumatoid Arthritis Derived Immune Complexes," *Arthritis & Rheumatism* 38 (1995): 744–49.

[12] L. Toohey, "Natural Substances Combat Arthritis with 'Immune power,'" *Nutri Notes* 2 (1997): 1–6.

[13] L. Cordain *et al.*, "Modulation of Immune Function by Dietary Lectins in Rheumatoid Arthritis," *British Journal of Nutrition* 83 (2000), 207–17.

[14] S. Parcell, "Biochemical and Nutritional Influences on Pain, Integrative Pain Medicine," *Contemporary Pain Medicine* (2008): 133–72.

[15] J. Visser *et al.*, "Tight Junctions, Intestinal Permeability, and Autoimmunity: Celiac Disease and Type 1 Diabetes Paradigms," *Annals of the New York Academy of Sciences* 1165 (2009): 195–205.

defense mechanism in a dysfunctional manner occurs, which manifests as an autoimmune disease.[16]

## Compared to What?

A few years ago I saw an Internet-based "true age" calculator that asked a variety of lifestyle questions to determine one's "true age" as opposed to chronological age. Some of the questions were obvious: How often do you exercise? Are you overweight? But other questions reflected a substantial lack of understanding, one of which was how many times a week you eat beans. The more times you ate beans, the healthier you were presumed to be.

There are a lot of studies that will declare various things to be healthy. Whole grains and beans are notable examples. But the important thing to keep in mind is that such declarations are *comparative.* That is, although eating (properly prepared) beans twice a week is likely to be more healthy than eating a large order of French fries at a burger joint, this only means they are *comparatively* beneficial rather than salutary in an absolute sense.

All such declarations are, by definition, comparative, including my own. Because we are all mortal and will ultimately pass from this world, we all have to die from something. Eventually, any mammal that lives long enough and doesn't die from something else will develop some form of cancer. So there's no getting out of this world alive.

Everyone has seen the stories of 100-year-old women celebrating their birthdays with a shot of whiskey and a cigar—declaring these to be the secret of their longevity. And we've likewise seen people struck down at an early age by inexplicable illness despite seemingly having done everything right to reduce risks.

In medical parlance, where no absolute causation exists, various dietary components or lifestyle choices are referred to as *risk factors.* The fact you are sedentary does not guarantee that you will die from a heart attack. The fact you smoke doesn't guarantee

---

[16] R. Hamid and A. Masood, "Dietary Lectins as Disease Causing Toxicants," *Pakistan Journal of Nutrition* 8, no. 3 (2009): 293–303.

that you will get lung cancer. The fact you drink alcohol doesn't guarantee that you'll get cirrhosis. You can increase your risks or decrease them, but you can never guarantee a particular outcome or completely eliminate risks.

The relevance of the foregoing to caveman diet is this: Caveman diet, in my opinion and based upon the research I will present, will increase your odds of a happy, healthy life free of chronic and autoimmune diseases. It will substantially increase your odds of a healthy life when compared with the standard Western diet as generally promulgated by the powers that be, but there are no guarantees.

# Chapter 3
# Why Legumes Should Come with a Warning Label

Almost all the books I've read on preagricultural diet have devoted a substantial amount of space to why you shouldn't eat grains but almost none on legumes with the exception of soy. Soy is low-hanging fruit. That is, it is easy to explain why you shouldn't eat soy. But why shouldn't you eat kidney beans?

Beans were a staple of my diet since childhood. I always enjoyed a big pot of pinto beans cooked with ham or bacon and a side of corn bread slathered with butter. That, to me, was a meal fit for a king. Unfortunately, the only healthy thing in that meal is the ham. Most people who adopt a caveman diet most sorely miss sugar or grain products, such as pasta. But for me, beans were the biggest change. And believe me, as much as I have always enjoyed them, I wouldn't have given them up without a really good reason.

As I mentioned briefly in the previous chapter, beans are generally seen as healthy for a variety of reasons: They contain fiber, they contain minerals, and they contain B vitamins. A number of studies show that eating beans is healthy. But, again, I will ask, compared to *what*? Taken as an absolute, beans are only a worthwhile addition to one's diet in order to avoid imminent starvation. Otherwise, they should be avoided because in the long term, they do you only harm and no good.

Beans contain a number of substances that make them unfit for human consumption. Among these substances are lectins, saponins, hormonal disruptors, and excessive phytates.

## Phytohaemagglutinin

Phytohaemagglutinin is a two-part lectin present in most varieties of beans. Its name, translated to English, means "something from a plant that makes blood stick together." Its two parts consist of PHA-L and PHA-E—the L-variety agglutinates leukocytes (the white blood cells that fight infection) and the E-variety agglutinates erythrocytes (the red blood cells that carry oxygen).

Beans need to be boiled for at least ten minutes at full boiling temperature to denature this toxin. Simple slow cooking at temperatures below boiling actually concentrates the toxin. As few as five raw kidney beans are sufficient to cause poisoning symptoms. When beans whose phytohaemagglutinin hasn't been denatured are consumed, the most common symptoms are nausea, vomiting, diarrhea, and abdominal pain. The poison, thankfully, stays confined to the gastrointestinal tract and will pass in time.

(This toxin is why, back when I ate beans, I usually made them in a pressure cooker at a temperature of 240°F.)

As a point of common sense, does it make sense to eat something that has to be handled like this in order to not be immediately poisonous? Maybe it makes sense when the alternative is more or less immediate starvation, but otherwise it would seem wise to avoid.

Unfortunately, this isn't the only problem with beans.

## Saponins

The term "saponin" is a catchall phrase meaning "soap-like." Saponins are not universally harmful, but they are in fact like soap and have many of the same properties, including the ability to cleanse the skin of oils. Many soaps are nontoxic, meaning if you get a bit in your mouth, you'll be okay. But what if you ate soap every day?

The biggest effect of saponins that you eat is that they make it easier for macromolecules (such as lectin proteins) to pass through the intestinal wall straight into your bloodstream. Four researchers summarize the results of their experiment:

> The results indicate that some saponins readily increase the permeability of the small intestinal mucosal cells, thereby inhibiting active nutrient transport, and facilitating the

uptake of materials to which the gut would normally be impermeable.[1]

Assuming the food you were eating was otherwise wholesome, eating some saponins wouldn't be a problem. But beans are not wholesome. They contain things you most assuredly do not want in your bloodstream, and the saponins in the beans help make sure they are absorbed.

## Endocrine Disruptors

Our endocrine system is very complex and includes self-regulating feedback loops for a number of hormones. Though our endocrine systems include all hormones made in the body—including corticosteroids, melatonin, thyroid hormones, and others—it is our sex hormones that come most readily to mind when we speak of the endocrine system.

Endocrine disruptors are defined to be substances that "interfere with the synthesis, secretion, transport, binding, action, or elimination of natural hormones in the body that are responsible for development, behavior, fertility, and maintenance of homeostasis (normal cell metabolism)."[2] Endocrine disruptors are also called xenohormones—meaning hormones (or substances that act like hormones) that originate outside the body.

Endocrine disruptors have medical applications, such as birth control, relieving symptoms of menopause, slowing the progress of hormone-sensitive cancers of the prostate and breast, assisting with gender reassignment, and (in some countries) chemical castration. The hormone disruptors used in medicine are, of course, pure compounds that have been well characterized and

---

[1] I. T. Johnson *et al.*, Influence of Saponins on Gut Permeability and Active Nutrient Transport In Vitro, *Journal of Nutrition* 116, no. 11 (1986): 2270–77.

[2] T. M. Crisp *et al.*, "Environmental Endocrine Disruption: An Effects Assessment and Analysis," *Environmental Health Perspectives* 106, suppl. 1 (1998): 11–56.

exhaustively studied. They are used in very specific dosages with an eye toward adverse drug interactions and balancing benefits against unwanted side effects.

But endocrine disruptors can have other (and usually undesired) effects, and this is especially the case when a gestating baby is exposed to them while still inside the mother. This is the time when the cells of a fertilized egg divide rapidly and differentiate to form every system of the body and mind. So this is where we are most vulnerable to the effects of endocrine disruptors.[3] Hormones provided by the mother during this stage of development—and the balance and timing of these hormones—profoundly affect the brain development of the child. But they can also have epigenetic effects[4] that will predispose a child to cancer, obesity, or other problems as adults.

When we think of endocrine disruptors, we are usually thinking of environmental chemicals, but the much-touted phytoestrogens in various foods, such as legumes, can have the same effects. Studies have raised concerns that a pregnant mother consuming genistein (present in soy and other foods) can predispose her female offspring to breast cancer[5] and male offspring to prostate cancer.[6]

In fact, the governments of Switzerland, Israel, and the U.K. have issued statements warning pregnant women against consuming soy products because of these and other adverse effects in babies. Of course, the U.K., Israel, and Switzerland don't have gigantic

---

[3] R. Bigsby *et al.*, "Evaluating the Effects of Endocrine Disruptors on Endocrine Function During Development," *Environmental Health Perspectives* 107, suppl. 4 (1994): 613–18.

[4] Epigenetic effects pertain not to the genes themselves but to whether those genes are turned on or off and the degree to which they are expressed. Epigenetic effects are a prime example of how environment can affect genetic expression.

[5] L. Hilakivi-Clarke *et al.*, "Maternal Exposure to Genistein During Pregnancy Increases Carcinogen-Induced Mammary Tumorigenesis in Female Rat Offspring," *Oncology Reports* 6, no. 5 (1999): 1089–95.

[6] R. Santti *et al.*, "Developmental Estrogenization and Prostatic Neoplasia," *Prostate* 24, no. 2 (1994): 67–78.

fields of genetically modified soy—or an equally gigantic soy industry and accompanying soy lobby—like the United States has.

Endocrine disruptors in substances we eat as food are far more complex than those used in medicine. As part of food, they are usually present with other compounds. Quite often—and this is especially true with the phytoestrogens in legumes—they aren't even directly present in the food. Instead, bacteria in the gut serve to convert a less biologically active isoflavone (daidzein) into an estrogen analog (S-equol).[7]

The reliance on gut bacteria makes it hard to predict the effects, because a person's genes, diet, and environment determine the species of bacteria in his or her gut. Approximately 50 to 60 percent of Asians[8] can convert the daidzen in legumes to S-equol[8] whereas only approximately 25 to 30 percent of Westerners can do so.[9]

Though a great deal of concern is expressed regarding insecticides and plasticizers as endocrine disruptors, the simple fact is that most people willingly consume them in substantial quantities in the form of soy products primarily but also in grains and other legumes. Though most of the press about phytoestrogens pertains to soy, these compounds are also present in other beans, as well as peas.[10]

Humans live in an extremely complex environment, and it is very difficult to definitively attribute a specific adverse outcome to a particular food. For example, low sperm count and erectile

---

[7] C. Atkinson, C. L. Frankenfeld, and J. W. Lampe. "Gut Bacterial Metabolism of the Soy Isoflavone Daidzein: Exploring the Relevance to Human Health." *Experimental Biology and Medicine* (Maywood) 230, no. 3 (2005): 155–70.

[8] K. B. Song *et al.*, "Prevalence of Daidzein-Metabolizing Phenotypes Differs Between Caucasian and Korean American Women and Girls," *The Journal of Nutrition* 136, no. 5 (2006): 1347–51

[9] I. R. Rowland *et al.*, "Interindividual Variation in Metabolism of Soy Isoflavones and Lignans: Influence of Habitual Diet on Equol Production by the Gut Microflora," *Nutrition and Cancer* 36, no. 1 (2000): 27–32.

[10] Y. Nakamura *et al.*, "Content and Composition of Isoflavonoids in Mature or Immature Beans and Bean Sprouts Consumed in Japan," *Journal of Health Science* 47 no. 4 (2001): 394–406.

dysfunction can be caused by obesity because fat cells in men turn more testosterone into estrogen.

But a bit of common sense is in order.

You can barely get through a day without encountering some form of advertising touting the benefits of phytoestrogens contained in soy and other foods. If these phytoestrogens are physiologically active in women, they would also be physiologically active in men. If they are sufficiently physiologically active to have the many claimed medically beneficial effects, they would likewise have risks of adverse effects. Whether these phytoestrogens would be a net benefit to men is an interesting question, but I think its worth noting that, other than as a prelude to gender reassignment, doctors do not prescribe estrogen to men. Though estrogen no doubt has lots of benefits and protective effects, it also comes with some downsides for men that most would rather avoid.

Studies are mixed. One of the reasons for this is that how biologically active the compounds in soy are for a given individual is determined to some degree by the person's gut bacteria.[11]

But consuming endocrine disruptors *without even realizing they are being consumed* and with no specific goal in doing so exposes you to all the effects without your knowledge. There is evidence that the isoflavones in soy reduce sperm count in men.[12] The fact that ads for erectile dysfunction medications are ubiquitous may also have something to do with the amount of soy in our diets, as a number of studies[13] indicate that consumption of soy can indeed cause impotence.

[11] C. Atkinson, C. L. Frankenfeld, and J. W. Lampe, "Gut Bacterial Metabolism of the Soy Isoflavone Daidzein: Exploring the Relevance to Human Health," *Experimental Biology and Medicine* (Maywood) 230, no. 3 (2005): 155–70.

[12] J. E. Chavarro *et al.*, "Soy Food and Isoflavone Intake in Relation to Semen Quality Parameters Among Men from an Infertility Clinic," *Human Reproduction* 23, no. 11 (2008): 2584–90.

[13] T. Siepmann *et al.*, "Hypogonadism and Erectile Dysfunction Associated with Soy Product Consumption," *Nutrition* 27, nos. 7–8 (2011): 859–62.

Of course women are no more immune than men. There is considerable data indicating that consuming the endocrine disruptors in legumes can impair a woman's fertility.[14] This isn't surprising when it's considered that plants developed phytoestrogens as a protective mechanism specifically to reduce the fertility of animals that eat them.[15, 16, 17]

As I pointed out earlier, though much of this attention is focused on soy, other legumes contain the same compounds although usually in lower quantities.

## Antinutrients

Legumes are high in phytic acid. Nearly all plants contain some amount of phytic acid, and considering that it can have anticancer properties,[18] it isn't a universally harmful substance. But as with many things, it is the *amount* that spells the difference between harmless and toxic. Someone with an excellent diet that is already very high in all essential nutrients can consume as much as 800 mg of phytic acid daily without ill effects, whereas someone with a more typical diet shouldn't consume more than 400 mg daily.[19]

---

[14] J. Seppen, "A Diet Containing the Soy Phytoestrogen Genistein Causes Infertility in Female Rats Partially Deficient in UDP Glucuronyltransferase," *Toxicology and Applied Pharmacology* 264, no. 3 (2012): 335–42.

[15] P. Ehrlich and P. H. Raven, "Butterflies and Plants: A Study of Coevolution," *Evolution* 18 (1964): 586–608.

[16] C. L. Hughes Jr., "Phytochemical Mimicry of Reproductive Hormones and Modulation of Herbivore Fertility by Phytoestrogens," *Environmental Health Perspectives* 78 (1988): 171–74.

[17] L. J. Guillette Jr. *et al.*, "Organization Versus Activation: The Role of Endocrine-Disrupting Contaminants (EDCs) During Embryonic Development in Wildlife," *Environmental Health Perspectives* 103, suppl. 7 (1995): 157–64.

[18] I. Vucenik and A. Shamsuddin, "Cancer Inhibition by Inositol Hexaphosphate ($IP_6$) and Inositol: From Laboratory to Clinic," *Journal of Nutrition* 133, no. 11 (2003): 3778S–3784S.

[19] R. Nagel, "Living with Phytic Acid," *Weston A. Price Foundation* March 26, 2010; available at www.westonaprice.org/food-features/living-with-phytic-acid.

It is important to note that we eat phytic acid without eating legumes, because both mammalian cells and plant cells make phytic acid as a store of phosphorus. But the amounts made in animal tissue and plant leaves are minuscule. Phytic acid tends to concentrate in the hulls of seeds. For example, broccoli contains 18 mg of phytic acid per 100 g, whereas pinto beans (a seed) contain 2,380 mg of phytic acid per 100 g. (As a point of reference, 100 g is a bit under 4 oz.)

Phytic acid is a powerful chelation agent. It combines with metallic and semimetallic elements, such as phosphorus, iron, and manganese, to form an insoluble precipitate that passes through the digestive tract and is eliminated in feces. It is such a powerful chelation agent that it is used to remove uranium in individuals so unfortunate as to be exposed. Though this chelation effect is medically useful on a short-term basis in treatment of heavy metal poisoning, on a long-term basis, especially for people whose diets are nutritionally poor, it is bad news.

Phytic acid combines with important minerals in the digestive tract and makes them unavailable for absorption. This includes iron (needed for red blood cells and oxygen transport), zinc (needed for the immune system and reproductive health), calcium (needed for heart and bone health), and magnesium (needed for brain and bone health), among others. A diet rich in legumes containing phytic acid can give rise to diseases caused by deficiency of these important minerals.[20, 21] It also combines with important B vitamins, such as niacin. For this reason, people following diets in which beans play a prominent role as a protein source usually have to cope with nutrient malabsorption problems.[22]

---

[20] R. F. Hurrell, "Influence of Vegetable Protein Sources on Trace Element and Mineral Bioavailability," *The Journal of Nutrition* 133, no. 9 (2003).

[21] Committee on Food Protection, Food and Nutrition Board, National Research Council, "Phytates," in *Toxicants Occurring Naturally in Foods*, ed. F. M. Strong (Washington, DC: National Academy of Sciences, 1973), 363–71.

[22] G. Famularo *et al.*, "Probiotic Lactobacilli: An Innovative Tool to Correct the Malabsorption Syndrome of Vegetarians?" *Medical Hypotheses* 65, no. 6 (2005): 1132–35.

## Protease Inhibitors

Protease is the generic term for any enzyme that breaks down food proteins into their constituent amino acids so they can be absorbed from the digestive tract.

Legumes contain protease inhibitors, which are compounds that prevent our digestive enzymes from doing their job. Though the protease inhibitors in legumes seem to have evolved primarily to defeat insect pests,[23] they nevertheless make as much as 50 percent of the protein in legumes unavailable via digestion.[24]

Considering that lectins present in beans are also proteins, the protease inhibitors also serve to keep those lectins intact so that they can do other damage. Though the lectin phytohaemagglutinin was mentioned earlier in the chapter, there are other lectins present that have been implicated in irritable bowel syndrome, arthritis, multiple sclerosis, and a number of other chronic diseases.[25]

## Indigestible Sugars and High Carbohydrate Content

Ounce for ounce, though beans will serve as a protein source if nothing else is available, they are a poor source of protein compared with meats. A cup of cooked kidney beans contains 15.2 g of proteins, whereas a six-ounce serving of dark meat chicken contains 47.2 g of protein.

On the other hand, legumes tend to be relatively high in carbohydrates, with as much as 30 g of available carbohydrates per serving. Though a caveman diet is not an explicitly "low carb" diet, given the otherwise problematic nutrition of legumes, the carbs in

---

[23] Y. Birk, "Protein Proteinase Inhibitors in Legume Seeds—Overview," *Archivos Latinoamericanos de Nutrición* 44, 4 suppl. 1 (1996): 26S–30S.

[24] G. S. Gilani, K. A. Cockell, and E. Sepehr, "Effects of Antinutritional Factors on Protein Digestibility and Amino Acid Availability in Foods," *Journal of AOAC International* 88, no. 3 (2005): 967–87.

[25] D. Freed, "Do Dietary Lectins Cause Disease?" *BMJ* 318, no. 7190 (1999), 1023–24.

beans don't come with enough nutritional value to justify their consumption.

But it is the indigestible sugars that pose the larger problem. Everyone knows that legumes cause flatulence. The indigestible oligosaccharides (an oligosaccharide is a chain of different types of sugars) of the raffinose family can't be digested, because mammals don't make an enzyme called $\alpha$-galactosidase. As a result, the oligosaccharides in beans pass into the large intestine, where they serve as food for anaerobic bacteria that generate gases responsible for flatulence.

Though flatulence may be a social issue, in and of itself it isn't a reason not to eat beans.

Your large intestine is its own specialized environment filled with all kinds of microorganisms that play a role in everything from your immune system[26] to your behavior.[27] Many environmental factors can influence which microbes are in your gut and in what proportions. One of the larger influences over which you have control is the food you provide. Just like their human hosts, intestinal bacteria have dietary preferences. The bacteria encouraged by these oligosaccharides can contribute to irritable bowel syndrome and other bowel problems.[28, 29]

## Can Legumes Be Consumed Safely?

Saponins are reduced by properly soaking beans before cooking. To properly soak beans, put them in a pot with three times

---

[26] K. Da Silva, "Gut Bugs Alter Antiviral Immunity," *Nature Medicine* 18, no. 8 (2012): 1193.

[27] K. Neufeld *et al.*, "Reduced Anxiety-like Behavior and Central Neurochemical Change in Germ-Free Mice," *Neurogastroenterology & Motility* 23 (2011).

[28] R. Goldstein, D. Braverman, and H. Stankiewicz, "Carbohydrate Malabsorption and the Effect of Dietary Restriction on Symptoms of Irritable Bowel Syndrome and Functional Bowel Complaints," *Israel Medical Association Journal* 2, no. 8 (2000): 583–87.

[29] W. Scheppach *et al.*, "Effect of Starch Malabsorption on Colonic Function and Metabolism in Humans." *Gastroenterology* 95, no. 6 (1988): 1549–55.

their volume of water, raise to boiling temperature for at least ten minutes (which also deactivates the phytohaemagglutinin), then cover and turn off the heat. Allow to sit for an hour, stir thoroughly, then pour off the liquid. Replace with fresh water before cooking.

It can be difficult to remove enough phytic acid from beans to make them safe. One method traditional cultures have used for reducing phytic acid content of legumes is sprouting. Sprouting legumes increases their phytase content, which in turn reduces the phytic acid and increases the bioavailability of minerals.[30] Another method is lactic acid fermentation.

One technique that can work on an industrial scale is holding the beans in aqueous solution at precisely 157 degrees for a sufficient period of time. The reason this would have to be done industrially is because the enzymes don't work at temperatures much lower than 157 degrees and are destroyed at 160 degrees, so the controls on a modern stove aren't sensitive enough to work.

The oligosaccharides can be dealt with by eating an enzyme product that will provide for their digestion or by consuming legumes along with a probiotic supplement containing Lactobacillus fermentum.

Though a tablespoon of cooked beans in a salad once in a while won't pose a risk to health, it should be clear from the above that in order to consume them safely as a dietary staple, they require extensive processing. Though this can make sense if other sources of protein are unavailable, meat can provide a lot more protein for considerably less effort.

---

[30] L. Camacho *et al.*, "Nutritional Changes Caused by the Germination of Legumes Commonly Eaten in Chile," *Archivos Latinoamericanos de Nutrición* 42, no. 3 (1992): 283–90.

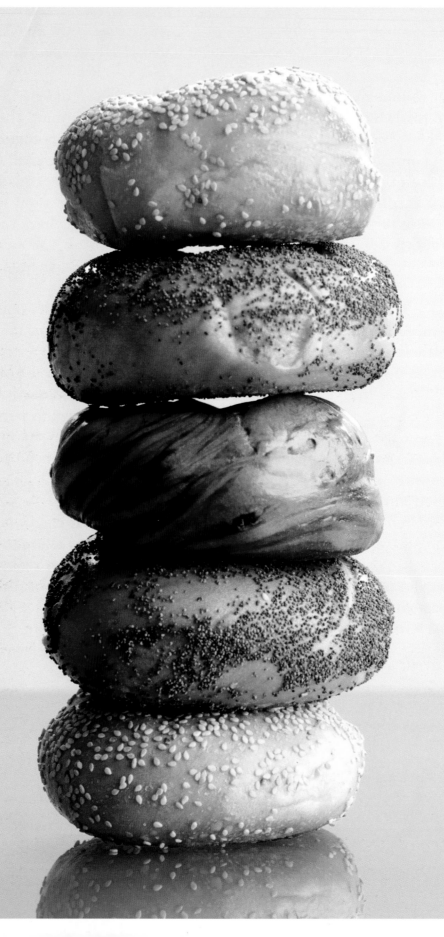

# Chapter 4
# Why You Should Avoid Grains Like the Plague

Grains are bad for you in so many ways that, comparatively speaking, they make beans look like health food. In fact, you are better off eating a spoonful of pure sugar than a slice of bread. Grains are really that bad.

Learning this was not good news for me. I love bread in all its myriad forms. For years before adopting a caveman diet, I made my own bread both as sourdough and in bread machines. For cultural reasons I have always loved biscuits and gravy. I whip up corn bread that causes ecstasy. My all-time favorite dessert is chocolate cake.

When I describe my diet to people, the first thing they ask me is if I miss grain products, but I can honestly say that I don't and that after my first two weeks without them, I have never had the slightest craving. Perhaps the reason for this is that the total elimination of grain from my diet turned out to be the key to recovering my health and well-being. I feel so well without it that I literally consider it to be poisonous.

I made a couple of errors on my path to eliminating grains. My first error was believing that unless you have full-blown celiac disease, grain is fine. My second error was in trying to eliminate only gluten and substituting a bunch of other novel grains (such as sorghum) in place of wheat. But when I finally eliminated *all* grains, within two weeks I felt better than I had in at least a decade. It was only with that experience that I finally realized just how badly I had been feeling.

I realize that grains form the foundation of the government-endorsed food pyramid and are also touted as being wonderful by various and sundry organizations. Maybe you like grains. Maybe you feel like you're doing just fine eating grains and "if it ain't broke, don't fix it." If you feel like that, it's worth keeping in mind that if you are like most Americans, you can't remember a single day of your life when you didn't eat grains, and while how you feel currently may seem normal to you, you really have nothing to compare against.

Given that every individual has followed a slightly different evolutionary path, it is certainly possible that you have evolved in such a way that grains are truly healthy for you. But I'd say the odds are against it. Read the case against grains, and decide for yourself.

## Grains Are Not Necessary

When Captain James Cook encountered the Aboriginal peoples of Australia, they had no farming or grain yet were perfectly healthy. This same pattern occurred with every hunter-gatherer people encountered by the seafaring explorers. Even when looking at modern hunter-gatherers without access to grain, such as the !Kung,[1] they are perfectly healthy.

The archaeological record is clear as well: While it is possible that there was sporadic access to grain prior to the dawn of agriculture, bone studies show that the protein source of early modern humans in the Paleolithic age was from animals.

The archaeological record is even clearer about the fact that the dawn of agriculture and reliance on grains brought about a decline in individual health in myriad ways.

Governments can lie, either deliberately or through innocent reliance on experts with an agenda. Likewise, people simply have a tendency to conform to dominant beliefs. Either way, the facts of archeology and thousands of years of human observation don't support the idea of grains being *necessary* for human health. The real question isn't whether they are necessary but whether they should be consumed at all.

---

[1] The exclamation point is used to denote a clicking sound in certain African "click languages." Many of these languages are in danger of extinction.

Even scientists are prone to blind acceptance in many cases. For example, I found a study in which an alpha amylase inhibitor was administered to dogs with their meals in order to keep the dogs from digesting carbohydrates so their diabetes could be controlled.[2] I looked at that study and wondered: Since dogs descended from wolves and are still so closely related they can interbreed, and since wolves have never run farms or raised grain, why on earth are you feeding grains to dogs in the first place? A great many pet foods for carnivores do indeed contain grains, and it can hurt them in myriad ways. If you have a cat or dog, I'd highly recommend visiting the website of veterinarian Dogtor J at dogtorj.com for some insight on what your pets should (and shouldn't) be eating.

## Grain: The Biggest Source of Tooth Decay

Again, the archaeological record is quite convincing. Prior to the adoption of grains, human beings simply did not have tooth decay.[3] Though I am sure sugar is a contributor as well, it should be understood that grains are a source of carbohydrates that are easily broken down into simple sugars.

If you are having a problem with cavities or believe you have "soft teeth" that are particularly vulnerable, switching to a modern caveman diet will solve the problem. You may still have problems with prior dental work or with existing cavities, but you won't be getting any new ones.

It was grain-based diets that brought the curse of ubiquitous dental problems down on our heads,[4] and undertaking a modern

---

[2] D. Koike, K. Yamadera, and E. P. DiMagno, "Effect of a Wheat Amylase Inhibitor on Canine Carbohydrate Digestion, Gastrointestinal Function, and Pancreatic Growth," *Gastroenterology* 108, no. 4 (1995): 1221–29.

[3] K. Gruber, "Oral Mystery: Are Agriculture and Rats Responsible for Tooth Decay?" *Scientific American*, February 6, 2013; available at www.scientificamerican.com/article.cfm?id=oral-mystery-are-agriculture-and-rates-responsible-for-tooth-decay.

[4] D. L. Greene, G. H. Ewing, and G. J. Armelagos, "Dentition of a Mesolithic Population from Wadi Halfa, Sudan," *American Journal of Physical Anthropology* 27 (1967): 41–55.

caveman diet from which grain is excluded will prevent and even heal cavities.[5,6]

If you don't consider getting your teeth drilled to constitute a fun time, just this fact alone should be a sufficient reason to eliminate grains from your diet. Unfortunately, this is only one of their most minor adverse effects.

## But I Must Have Fiber (from Grains) or I'll Die from Constipation!

Do you remember in the first chapter where I referenced the problem of conformity in medical science? Let me ask some questions. Why didn't our caveman ancestors without access to grain die from constipation? Why don't wolves, bears, and foxes all perish from exploding colons they couldn't evacuate? Why don't our genetically closest primate cousins, the great apes, die from constipation because of their failure to cultivate grain and eat bagels?

Let me ask another question. Why is it that with an entire aisle of the grocery store dedicated to cereals, and with most of them extolling the virtues of the fiber they contain, the very constipation grains are alleged to prevent constitutes the single most prevalent digestive complaint in the country?[7]

Though I will expand a bit more on the topics of fats and cholesterol in a later chapter, the factors causing constipation are the very things most promoted by our medical establishment. It's not a conspiracy, and it isn't maliciously intended. It's just that they blindly accept a variety of data from other experts—usually drug companies—and then pass it along as though it is unquestionable.

---

[5] W. Price, *Nutrition and Physical Degeneration* (La Mesa, CA: Price-Pottenger Nutrition, 2008).

[6] R. Nagel, *Cure Tooth Decay*: Heal And Prevent Cavities With Nutrition—Limit and Avoid Dental Surgery and Fluoride, 2d ed. (Ashland, OR: Golden Child Publishing, 2010).

[7] A. Sonnenberg and T. R. Koch, "Epidemiology of Constipation in the United States," *Diseases of the Colon & Rectum* 32, no. 1 (1989): 1–8.

If you are truly concerned about constipation—and odds are that you are because constipation or other bowel problems affect most adults in one way or another—then I suggest you should add a nice prime rib to your diet and ditch grain altogether. That is because the largest causes of constipation we are facing today is a lack of fat in the diet, overstimulation by fiber leading to the colon needing that stimulation in order to operate, and statin drugs.

Schmidt and Thews noted in *Human Physiology*, "Energy-rich meals with a high fat content increase motility [propulsion of stools]; carbohydrates and proteins have no effect."[8]

The mechanism by which fats prevent constipation is indirect but a fascinating study in the wonders of the body. Proteins (at least ideally) aren't absorbed directly into the bloodstream from the small intestine. Instead, they are broken up into their constituent amino acids by protease enzymes. The same thing happens with fats. When you eat some fat, as with the example of prime rib, the fats aren't absorbed directly into your body. Instead, they are broken up into their constituent fatty acids by bile made by the liver and secreted from the gall bladder. It is these fatty acids that are absorbed rather than the actual fat that was consumed.

Bile is secreted only in response to the presence of fat. Once enough has been secreted into the small intestine, the gastrocolic reflex is triggered. The gastrocolic reflex stimulates peristalsis (the movement of food through the intestines), which in turn stimulates defecation. This is the normal way defecation is stimulated in a healthy person. You'll know your large intestine is working the way it should when you are defecating at least once daily, usually soon after a meal. Two or more instances per day are more typical.

Dietary fats aren't the only way to stimulate defecation. Defecation can also be stimulated by sheer bulk of materials, irritation of the intestinal lining, or the accumulation of liquid in the intestines.

In the parlance of pharmaceuticals, laxatives that work by irritating the intestinal lining are called stimulant laxatives. Such

---

[8] R.F. Schmidt and G. Thews. "Colonic Motility," *Human Physiology*, 2d ed. (New York: Springer-Verlag, 1989), 731.

laxatives cause the intestinal lining to secrete large amounts of mucus to protect itself. A downside of intestinal irritants is that they are addictive.[9] No, they aren't addictive in the same sense as heroin. Rather, if used too often, your intestines become desensitized to normal stimulation and actually require the stimulation provided by an irritant in order to initiate defecation. Fiber is, in fact, both an irritant/stimulant[10] and a bulk[11] laxative.

So what occurs is a classic chicken-and-egg scenario. People eating grain-based diets rich in indigestible fibers create a situation in which their intestines become dependent on that stimulation in order to work properly. Since many people who emphasize grains in their diet (especially grains containing lots of fiber) are also conscientious about fats, the normal triggering method for defecation through bile doesn't occur.

To make matters even worse, many Americans, especially older Americans, are on salt-restricted diets. The body absorbs salt from the colon. If the amount of salt in the diet is insufficient, then the body sucks water out of the colon in order to recover what little precious salt it can. This leaves the stools hard as a rock and very difficult to pass. (I will address salt and our unreasoning paranoia of this essential substance in a later chapter.)

Meanwhile, constipation is one of the most common side effects of the ubiquitously prescribed statin drugs. When you consider that many older Americans are on fat-restricted and high-fiber diets combined with statins, is it at all surprising how many are also taking stool softeners?

Constipation is a problem that *wouldn't even exist* in the first place were it not for our heavily grain-based diets, the misguided

---

[9] W. S. Pray, "The Dilemma of the Patient Addicted to Stimulant Laxatives," *US Gastroenterology Review*, 2006; available at www. docstoc.com/docs/109579509/The-Dilemma-of-the-Patient-Addicted-to-Stimulant-Laxatives.

[10] "Scientists Learn More About How Roughage Keeps You 'Regular,'" *Since Daily*, August 23, 2006.

[11] R. F. Schmidt and G. Thews, "Colonic Motility," *Human Physiology*, 2d ed. (New York: Springer-Verlag, 1989).

war against fats, and a dependence on antibiotics and other drugs that adversely affect our intestines.

When people switch to a caveman diet, the volume of their fecal output tends to be reduced. This is normal. A caveman diet predominantly contains components that are completely broken down in the small intestine and thus never make it to the colon. So it is expected that someone on a caveman diet will make smaller bowel movements. As long as the movements are indeed regular, there is no cause for worry!

Incidentally, if you are concerned about the role fiber plays in preventing diabetes and cancer, if you actually read the studies, you'll find that these studies are referring to *vegetable* fiber. That is, they are referring to the fibers you get from eating your broccoli. Rest assured, a caveman diet has plenty of vegetables and plenty of nonirritating fiber.

## Antinutrients

The biggest antinutrient in grain is the same as with legumes: phytic acid. And just as with legumes, the phytic acid content of whole grains (the ones alleged to be the most healthy) is off the charts. As you'll recall, the phytic acid consumption of someone with an otherwise exemplary diet should be limited to 800 mg per day, and for people with a more typical diet it should be limited to 400 mg per day. Exceeding these thresholds on an ongoing basis risks deficiencies in vital minerals. Brown rice has 940 mg of phytic acid, rye contains 1,010 mg, and wheat can contain as much as 1,350 mg. Just three dry ounces of any grain contain more phytic acid than can be safely consumed.

Unfortunately, grains are not consumed in modest quantities in the typical American diet. In keeping with USDA recommendations, between six and eleven servings daily are the norm. I remember when I used to eat grains, I would heap my plate full of pasta, smother it in sauce, and have garlic bread on the side. As a result, the impact of antinutrients is quite real. Phytic acid in grains binds to important minerals, such as iron and zinc, making them completely unavailable so they are passed in the stool. So eating spinach alongside your whole-grain pasta can have the effect of making the iron from that spinach unavailable. You may have plenty of iron in your diet but suffer from deficiency anyway.

## Digestion Inhibitors

Grains are seeds. As such, their evolutionary intent, if eaten, is to pass through the gut intact and be deposited along with feces as fertilizer so they'll grow. In order to achieve this objective, grains contain digestion inhibitors.

Each type of grain contains slightly different compounds. There are so many, it would be pointless to name them all. For example, rice contains seventeen compounds that inhibit trypsin (the enzyme that digests protein in the small intestine),[12] while barley has twenty-two.[13]

Some grains, such as wheat, also contain alpha-amylase inhibitors, which prevent the breakdown of starches into their constituent sugars. These enzymes are destroyed by heat so they don't figure into dietary concerns. But while researching this book, I found an interesting study[14] in which scientists were researching using the alpha-amylase inhibitors in wheat to treat diabetes in humans. The idea was to make it so the carbohydrates couldn't be digested into their constituent sugars. The reason why humans are eating grains in the first place was not discussed.

This is a classic case of humans following the recommendations of scientists to eat grains, those recommendations resulting in the

[12] A. Singh, C. Sahi, and A. Grover, "Chymotrypsin Protease Inhibitor Gene Family in Rice: Genomic Organization and Evidence for the Presence of a Bidirectional Promoter Shared Between Two Chymotrypsin Protease Inhibitor Genes," *Gene* 428, nos. 1–2 (2009): 9–19.

[13] L. C. Bruhn and R. Djurtoft, "Protease Inhibitors in Barley," *Zeitschrift für Lebensmittel-Untersuchung und Forschung* 164, no. 4 (1977): 247–54.

[14] D. Piasecka-Kwiatkowska *et al.*, "Digestive Enzyme Inhibitors from Grains as Potential Components of Nutraceuticals," *Journal of Nutritional Science and Vitaminology* (Tokyo) 58, no. 3 (2012): 217–20.

horrible outcome of diabetes, and then the scientists riding to the rescue with a solution (undoubtedly a very expensive one) that never even questions the validity of their initial recommendation.

## Grain Lectins: Destroyers of Health

Lectins were described in an earlier chapter, but when it comes to grains, some more specifics are in order. Grains contain a number of lectins to which humans are not well adapted. For example, wheat germ agglutinin binds to insulin receptors and displaces insulin.[15] When this happens, blood glucose isn't metabolized as usual.

Grain lectins also cause leptin resistance.[16] Though many people have heard of insulin resistance, leptin resistance isn't a household term. Leptin is a hormone that signals satiety. It inactivates hormones that tell you that you are hungry and tells you it is time to stop eating. As you can probably imagine, if the receptors for leptin become resistant to its influence, the outcome is severe overeating and obesity—usually morbid obesity. You may notice that ever since we've been told how important it is that we eat as much as eleven servings of grain daily, rates of morbid obesity in this country have skyrocketed.

Grain lectins also bond to the inside of intestinal walls, mesangial cells, and the tubules in kidneys. They also activate HLA antigens on cells where those antigens aren't usually activated, particularly in the pancreas and thyroid.[17] In binding to the inside of intestinal walls, lectins actively damage the delicate epithelial tissues[18] as well as strip mucus from the intestinal lining. This

---

[15] P. Cuetrecasas and G. Tell, "Insulin-Like Activity of Concanavalin A and Wheat Germ Agglutinin—Direct Interactions with Insulin Receptors," *Proceedings of the National Academy of Sciences of the United States of America* 70, no. 2 (1973): 485–89.

[16] T. Jonsson *et al.*, "Agrarian Diet and Diseases of Affluence—Do Evolutionary Novel Dietary Lectins Cause Leptin Resistance?" *BMC Endocrine Disorders* 5 (2005): 10.

[17] D. Freed, "Do Dietary Lectins Cause Disease?" *BMJ* 318 (1999): 1023–24.

[18] K. Miyake, T. Tanaka T, and P. L. McNeil, "Lectin-Based Food Poisoning: A New Mechanism of Protein Toxicity," *PLoS ONE* 2, no. 8 (2007): e687.

opens up the bloodstream to direct invasion by food particles and compounds that were never intended to be in our bloodstream, triggering inflammation and an immune response.

The book *Plant Lectins* describes unhealthy lectins in unflattering terms.

> High degree of resistance to gut proteolysis. Binding to brush border cells; damage to microvillus membrane; shedding of cells; reduction in the absorptive capacity of the small intestine. Increased endocytosis; induction of hyperplastic growth of the small intestine; increased turnover of epithelial cells. Interference with the immune system; hypersensitivity reactions. Interference with the microbial ecology of the gut; selective overgrowth. Direct and indirect effects (hormones, etc.) on systemic metabolism.[19]

In short, the lectins in grains are a disaster for the human body. Though some people can handle them better than others, I recommend not eating them at all, since grains are by no means necessary for our health.

## Gluten

Though some other grains contain gluten, gluten-containing grains that we are most likely to encounter are wheat, rye, and barley. Gluten is the protein that makes wheat such a delight for making breads, but it is also a source of serious problems for many people.

A small percentage of people have celiac disease. Celiac disease is an autoimmune disease in which consumption of gluten leads the body to attack the microvilli in the small intestine. Abstention from gluten alleviates the disease.

If that were the whole story, it wouldn't be very important. What is more interesting is that even though few people are celiacs, a

---

[19] A. Pusztai, *Plant Lectins* (New York: Cambridge University Press, 1992).

large portion of the population is sensitive to gluten. By "sensitive" I mean that in testing stool samples, 29 percent of completely asymptomatic people are producing antibodies against one of the proteins in gluten; 62 percent of people with autoimmune diseases are positive for the antibodies; 57 percent of people with digestive problems are positive for gluten antibodies.

At best, then, there is a 29 percent chance that you are sensitive to gluten, but the odds are greatly increased if you have any autoimmune disease or digestive problem. A review in the *New England Journal of Medicine* listed fifty-five diseases thought to be caused in whole or in part by exposure to gluten.[20]

The production of antibodies against gluten indicates that, at some point, whether due to damage to the intestinal lining from lectins or from fiber, the gluten proteins actually made it into the bloodstream. Are the 71 percent of people who don't produce the antibodies fully adapted to gluten? Or are they just lucky so far in that gluten hasn't entered their bloodstream?

The answer to that question lies in the genes, or to be very specific, a gene named HLA-DQ. This gene can be encoded eight different ways, only one of which is completely adapted to gluten. Only 0.4 percent of the U.S. population carries that specific encoding for HLA-DQ and no other. So the odds against gluten being something you should eat are 99.6 percent.[21] In fact, the longer you eat gluten, the more likely you are to develop an autoimmune disease, including rheumatoid arthritis, psoriasis, lupus, celiac disease and others.[22] So when it comes to eating grains containing

---

[20] R. Farrell and C. Kelley, "Celiac Sprue," *New England Journal of Medicine* 346, no. 3 (2002): 180–88.

[21] C. Zanchi *et al.*, "Bone Metabolism in Celiac Disease," *Journal of Pediatrics* 153, no.2 (2008): 262–65.

[22] V. Petersen, "Is Gluten Intolerance the Cause of Autoimmune Disease?" *Health Now Medical Center*, July 5, 2011; available at www.healthnow-medical.com/blog/2011/07/05/is-gluten-intolerance-the-cause-of-auto-immune-disease/.

gluten, you are playing the odds. To paraphrase a famous movie character, you have to ask yourself, "Do you feel lucky?"

## Concentrated Carbohydrates

Grains are a store of concentrated carbohydrates. Carbohydrates are simply long strings of sugar molecules bound together. When the carbohydrates encounter digestive enzymes, they are broken up into simple sugars that are directly absorbed into the bloodstream.

Our bodies contain numerous enzymes, such as ptyalin and amylase, that are intended to break down carbohydrates and are able to directly absorb simple sugars. It is clear that our evolutionary background is compatible with consuming carbohydrates and simple sugars to some degree.

But "to some degree" doesn't mean we evolved for carbohydrates to be the very core and foundation of our diet! I will expand more on carbohydrates and the quantities of carbohydrates that are healthy in our diet in a later chapter, and for now I will put the concentration of carbohydrates present in grains into perspective.

Looking at the label of a widely available organic multigrain bread, two slices (enough to make a sandwich) provide 40 g of carbohydrate. A teaspoon of sugar contains 4 g of carbohydrate. So those two slices of organic multigrain bread contain as much carbohydrate as ten teaspoons of sugar. And, the only difference between eating pure glucose and the most "healthy" and "slowly broken down" of grain-based carbs is that the latter won't hit your bloodstream until about forty minutes later than the former.

You are probably aware of the big deal being made about banning soft drinks over a certain size in schools and so forth because of the belief that the high amount of sugar in soda contributes to obesity. Well, it certainly *does* contribute to obesity. A twelve-ounce can of the best-selling name-brand cola contains 39 g of sugar. But a sandwich made with two slices of multigrain bread contains 42 g of carbohydrates that will turn into sugar within minutes of reaching the small intestine. The glycemic load for the two slices of bread is even higher than for the soft drink. (I explain glycemic load in greater depth in chapter 7.) Because of this, the bread from the sandwich has the same effect on insulin, blood glucose, and obesity as the soft drink. That doesn't sound like any sort of healthy food.

## But If I *Must* Eat Grain, Which Is Healthiest?

There is no reason why anyone in the United States *must* eat grain outside of a lifeboat survivalist scenario, and anyone with the leisure to read this book probably isn't in such a scenario. But since many people have asked me this question, I'll share my analysis.

Gluten-containing grains are out. The odds are against you being one of the 0.4 percent who can never develop an adverse reaction to gluten. So the following grains should always be avoided: barley, rye, wheat, spelt, kamut, and their derivatives, including bulgur, durum, semolina, farina, and graham.

This leaves us the following grains from which to choose: corn, millet, oats, rice, sorghum, and teff. Of these, only millet and sorghum haven't been demonstrated to have lectin activity.

Even though neither millet nor sorghum contains gluten per se, the prolamines in millet can cross-react in anyone already sensitized to gluten. Since 29 percent of people who are utterly asymptomatic demonstrate antibodies to gluten, your odds of cross-reacting with millet are twice as bad as with Russian roulette. If you have a history of digestive problems or autoimmune disease, your odds are even worse. So that leaves sorghum. That still doesn't solve the carbohydrate issue, but it addresses the problems with gluten and lectins.

A related question is: Can grains be made safe or safer? The answer is yes. Gluten-containing grains can't be made safe without completely destroying any food value they have. So going back to corn, millet, oats, rice, sorghum, and teff—they can all be made a lot safer in terms of antinutrients and lectins by employing the treatments used in traditional cultures around the world.

The phytic acid in most seeds can be removed by sprouting. To sprout, soak the seed in water overnight, drain, then gently rinse with water and drain twice daily thereafter until a sprout has grown that is twice as long as the seed. By that point, the seed has generated and employed enzymes that have destroyed all of the antinutrients.

The lectins require a follow-up phase: fermentation. Most traditional cultures use a lactic acid type of fermentation, but a process more akin to sourdough has been shown to be effective. All you do is soak the sprouted grain for twenty-four hours at room temperature in an open pot, then pour off the soaking water and cook in fresh water. The twenty-four hours spent at room temperature allow native bacteria in the air to take hold, and their enzymatic activity will assist in degrading the lectins.

Every time you do this, save a bit of the soaking water in the refrigerator, and add it back to the next batch. This will serve as a "starter" just as in sourdough. By the time you've made your third batch, the bacterial cultures will be strong enough that lectin and antinutrient degradation will be substantial.

So, yes, it is *possible* to make nongluten grains safe to eat. But it is also quite an involved process that isn't used in any commercially manufactured products and is a pain to do at home.

That having been said, a bit of popcorn when you go to the movies won't kill you. Popcorn actually uses a very small quantity of corn, and so far the specific varieties of corn used to make popcorn haven't been genetically modified. It's still bad for you in that it contains bad stuff, but so long as it is limited, don't sweat it. A big bowl of popcorn uses as many corn kernels as about one-third of an ear of corn. Live a little!

Plain white rice is also free of lectins and antinutrients because they are in the germ that is removed by polishing. It's still a concentrated carbohydrate, but one of the safer ones.

## How About Nongrain Grains?

This category refers to seeds that are used like grains for culinary purposes but aren't grains in a botanical sense. This includes buckwheat, quinoa, and amaranth. Buckwheat, quinoa, and amaranth are seeds, and as such they all have high phytic acid levels. They also have saponins (as described in the chapter on legumes) and lectins.

Making them safe to eat is a monumental undertaking incompatible with modern lifestyles. For example, to make quinoa safe for daily eating in substantial quantities it must first be sprouted, then dried and ground into flour. The flour must then be fermented for three days using a Lactobacillus plantarum starter culture, and then it is finally cooked. At that point you have a super high carb food-like product that generates insulin resistance and is helpful in the achievement of one's lifelong goals of becoming morbidly obese and diabetic.

I realize that there is a tendency to try to replicate all the foods people enjoyed before switching to a caveman diet, but in practice what I recommend is simply accepting a diet of real food and enjoying it abundantly.

Let me put it somewhat differently.

Later on in the chapter on carbohydrates, I'm going to explain that, in practice, you'll be limiting carbs to 20 to 25 percent of your calories. These calories will come mostly from fruits and vegetables. But you're allowed to cheat once in a while and splurge on something decadently sweet.

Pretend that you have just finished a rough workout on one of your cheat days and you need some fast carb calories. You can have those carb calories in the form of a small piece of sinfully decadent flourless chocolate cake or quinoa gruel that you have sprouted for three days, fermented for three days, and then boiled. Which do you choose? Seems like a no-brainer to me.

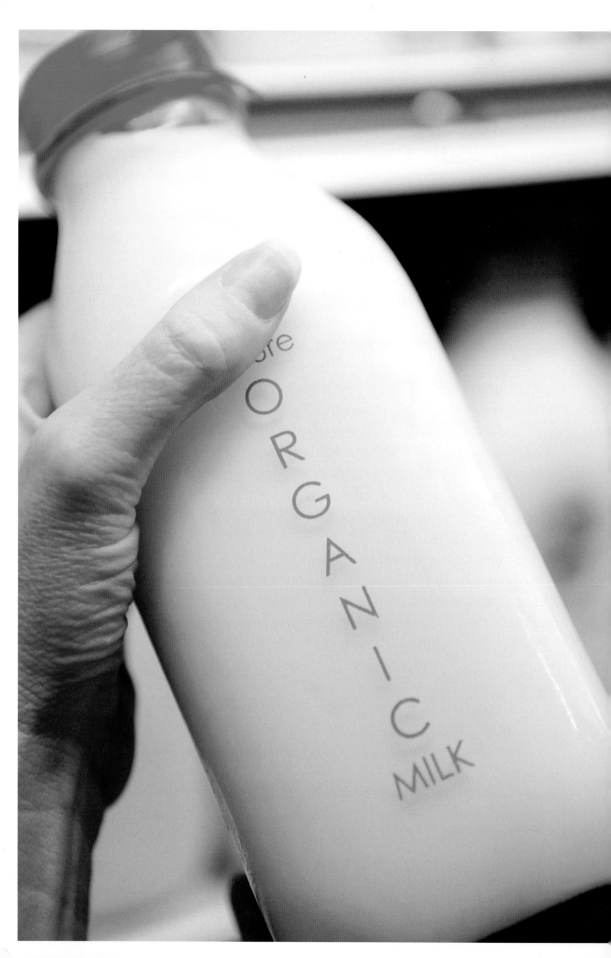

# Chapter 5
# Does Milk Do Your Body Good?

As a young elementary school student in the mid 1970s, I remember being treated to a TV program at school called *Mulligan Stew*. The purpose of the program was to teach nutrition, and it drilled the formula "4–4–3–2" into my head and the heads of my fellow students. The numbers reflected the USDA dietary guidelines of the time: You should have four servings of bread/cereal, four servings of fruits/vegetables, three servings of dairy, and two servings of meat, fish, or fowl daily in order to remain healthy.

The indoctrination was certainly effective because I remember pestering my parents to make sure I had three servings of dairy daily so I wouldn't sicken and perish from diseases stemming from nutritional deficiency. Naturally, as a well-trained nine-year-old, I was blissfully unaware at the time that the overwhelming proportion of humans on the planet are lactose intolerant[1] and thus unable to consume most dairy products in useful quantities without experiencing severe gastrointestinal distress and pain.

Because I was unaware of this fact and the teachers never mentioned it, I never asked the logical question: How is it that a substance that would literally make most humans acutely ill if they were to consume it must literally be *necessary* for my health according to the government? (At the time I was not aware of the concept of a lobbyist or a dairy subsidy either.)

Because I was never much of a milk drinker as an adult, I didn't even realize I was lactose intolerant until my mid thirties. Because hard cheeses are very low in lactose (the lactose is removed along with the whey during the initial stages of making cheese), they didn't give me a problem. I wasn't big into yogurt because it was too

---

[1] D. M. Swallow, "Genetics of Lactase Persistence and Lactose Intolerance," *Annual Review of Genetics* 37 (2003): 197–219

sweet, but sauces made from whole milk posed a problem for me. At first it seemed mysterious. I couldn't figure out why I had the embarrassing problem of passing gas constantly whenever I made my famous Alfredo sauce. Eventually, though, as the symptoms became more pronounced and obvious—culminating in my actually vomiting upon the ingestion of some buttermilk—I figured it out. As they say in New England, "dawn breaks over Marblehead."

Once I started researching lactose intolerance, that was the first thing that led me to question our food pyramid. How on earth could something be *essential* for my health if it would literally make me sick?

Of course, I am sure lactose intolerance never crossed the minds of my elementary school teachers as they plopped me in front of *Mulligan Stew* for my dose of government-approved indoctrination. Lactase persistence, that is, the ability to digest lactose into adulthood, doesn't exist in any mammals except humans. And it doesn't exist in all humans. In fact, it is a genetic adaptation that only came into existence during the past 10,000 years for a small portion of humanity.

Furthermore, the requisite genetic adaptations only exist broadly in population groups that tamed cattle and started drinking milk and making cheeses. This genetic adaptation is very common among people of European ancestry, but it is decidedly uncommon among East Asian populations. In fact, while between 85 and 95 percent of British adults can digest lactose without difficulty, somewhere between 90 and 100 percent of East Asian adults and between 70 and 90 percent of African adults can't digest lactose.[2]

Among descendants of dairying cultures, whenever lactose intolerance exists, it tends to be mild so that butter, hard cheeses, or a bit of cream can be consumed without difficulty. At the time I watched the several episodes of *Mulligan Stew*, I was living in Hickory, North Carolina, where nearly everyone at the time was of British or other European descent. Therefore, my teachers took it

---

[2] Michael de Vrese, "Probiotics: Compensation for Lactase Insufficiency," *American Journal of Clinical Nutrition* 73, no. 2 (2001).

for granted that everyone could drink the requisite three cups of milk daily without trouble.

My teachers were not alone. As recently as the 1960s, the Western medical community—demonstrating an amazing degree of ethnocentric nearsightedness—did not recognize lactose intolerance as a real condition. The symptoms of lactose intolerance were instead attributed to some sort of intestinal pathogen, an allergic reaction, or even (and I'm not kidding) psychosomatic causes.[3,4] This should be food for thought.

Mammals are born with the ability to digest lactose so they can derive sustenance from their lactating mothers. The milk passes along, between mammals of the same species anyway, a host of important factors besides sustenance, including immunity to various diseases. The benefits to children fed breast milk during their first months of life are both broad and dramatic. Children who are breast-fed until at least six months old have decreased risks of certain cancers,[5] decreased risk of obesity,[6] and superior gut flora that reduces the risks of infections and other illnesses.[7]

But all mammals lose the ability to digest lactose shortly after weaning, with the exception of a minority of humans (looking at *global* populations) who acquired adaptations that allow them to produce the enzymes for digesting lactose into adulthood. Whether milk (particularly from another animal species) is actively harmful

[3] S. Auricchio *et al.*, "Isolated Intestinal Lactase Deficiency in the Adult," *Lancet* 280 (1963): 324–26.

[4] F. J. Simoons, "Primary Adult Lactose Intolerance and the Milking Habit: A Problem in Biological and Cultural Interrelations," *Digestive Diseases and Sciences* 14, no. 12 (1969): 819–36.

[5] A. Bener, S. Denic, and S. Galadari, "Longer Breast-Feeding and Protection Against Childhood Leukaemia and Lymphomas," *European Journal of Cancer* 37, no. 2 (2001): 234–38.

[6] M. W. Gillman *et al.*, "Risk of Overweight Among Adolescents Who Were Breastfed as Infants," *Journal of the American Medical Association* 285, no. 19 (2001): 2461–67.

[7] Duke University Medical Center, "Breast Milk Promotes a Different Gut Flora Than Infant Formulas," *DukeHealth.org*, August 27, 2012; available at www.dukehealth.org/health_library/news/breast-milk-promotes-a-different-gut-flora-growth-than-infant-formulas.

or not is something we'll explore shortly. The point I am getting across is that the USDA guidelines I was taught as a child have *no rational scientific basis*. It makes absolutely no sense, considering that most people on the planet can't even drink milk without becoming ill, to put forward guidelines specifying its consumption as a prerequisite for health. So these guidelines merit serious scrutiny.

## Milk Is Not Necessary for Health

As I have already mentioned, the overwhelming preponderance of people on the planet can't even drink milk. A taste for fermented foods, such as cheeses, is culturally acquired, and many people from cultures without a history of dairy herding find even the aroma of cheese disgusting. Furthermore, the ability to consume milk has only come into our genome in the past 10,000 years.

The reason I am stressing this point is that there are a lot of debates about pasteurized versus unpasteurized, bovine growth hormone, antibiotics, organic, grass-fed, and so forth. Each side has some very interesting points. But these debates are not and cannot be over whether you *must* consume milk to be healthy. You absolutely positively do not *need* it in any form. The real question being addressed by these debates is whether you should consume milk products optionally at all, and if so, which types are most healthful or least harmful.

## But I Will Die from Osteoporosis as My Bones Crumble to Dust!

You can't believe everything someone in authority or with an air of expertise says. It's wise to apply a bit of common sense and ask a few questions. Does any other mammal die from osteoporosis because of its failure to regularly consume the milk of some other mammalian species into adulthood? Of course not. Is there any evidence that humans are somehow different? No. During the age of William Dampier, many cultures with no dairy herding were encountered, and they were uniformly perfectly healthy.

A while back I wrote a book on vegetable gardening. One of the things I highlighted for each vegetable was its nutritional content. It turns out that fruits and vegetables have plenty of calcium. A cup of skim milk has 300 mg of calcium. An ounce of most hard cheeses has 200 mg of calcium. Drinking three cups of skim milk daily would yield 900 mg of calcium.

A cup of cooked broccoli has 180 mg of calcium. A cup of spinach has 240 mg of calcium. Three ounces of turnip greens have 190 mg of calcium. A cup of okra has 170 mg of calcium. You get the idea. If you eat anywhere near as many vegetables as you should be eating, you will get more than enough calcium in your diet.

Fish, especially fish canned with the bones, is also high in calcium. A can of sardines yields 240 mg of calcium, and a cup of canned salmon has over 800 mg of calcium. Fresh fish can also provide a lot of calcium, with walleyed pike delivering 170 mg of calcium per fillet and a fillet of herring serving up 150 mg of calcium.

In other words, our ancestors from over 10,000 years ago, who had no adaptations that allowed them to drink milk and had not yet learned herding, got by just fine, and you can too. You need have no fear of osteoporosis simply from not drinking milk.

In fact, milk consumption in adults seems to have the opposite effect from what we'd expect. The conclusion of one study was pretty sobering: "Consumption of dairy products, particularly at age twenty years, was associated with an increased risk of hip fracture in old age."[8] The Harvard Nurse's Study, which followed 77,000 women for twelve years, concluded, "These data do not support the hypothesis that higher consumption of milk or other food sources of calcium by adult women protects against hip or

---

[8] R. G. Cumming and R. J. Klineberg, "Case-Control Study of Risk Factors for Hip Fractures in the Elderly," *American Journal of Epidemiology* 139, no. 5 (1994): 493–503.

forearm fractures."[9] Even adolescent girls who drink a lot of milk are at increased risk of stress fractures.[10]

If you are concerned about bone density, there are two things that have an unshakable proven track record of increasing bone density: weight-bearing progressive-resistance exercise[11,12,13,14] and eating a variety of fruits and vegetables.[15]

## Raw Versus Pasteurized Milk

It is said that milk is nature's most perfect food. And it is. Human milk is perfect for human babies. Cow's milk is perfect for calves who have four stomachs and grow to weigh 600 lbs before weaning. But the real question is: Is cow's milk perfect for adult humans?

The answer to this question is, unfortunately, not completely clear because there is a lot of confusion and not a lot of science to clarify that confusion. At the heart of the confusion is the difference between pasteurized and raw milk. Though there is a great deal of science indicating that the typical milk available at the

[9] D. Feskanich et al., "Milk, Dietary Calcium, and Bone Fractures in Women: A 12-Year Prospective Study," American Journal of Public Health (1997).

[10] K. R. Sonneville et al., "Vitamin D, Calcium, and Dairy Intakes and Stress Fractures Among Female Adolescents," Archives of Pediatrics and Adolescent Medicine 166, no. 7 (2012): 595–600.

[11] M. Lunt et al., "The Effects of Lifestyle, Dietary Dairy Intake and Diabetes on Bone Density and Vertebral Deformity Prevalence: The EVOS Study," Osteoporos International 12 (2001): 688–98.

[12] S. Going et al., "Effects of Exercise on Bone Mineral Density in Calcium-Replete Postmenopausal Women with and without Hormone Replacement Therapy," Osteoporos International 4, no. 8 (2003): 637–43.

[13] R. Prince et al., "The Effects of Calcium Supplementation (Milk Powder or Tablets) and Exercise on Bone Mineral Density in Postmenopausal Women," Journal of Bone and Mineral Research 10 (1995): 1068–75.

[14] T. Lloyd et al., "Modifiable Determinants of Bone Status in Young Women," Bone 30 (2002): 416–21.

[15] K. L. Tucker et al., "Potassium, Magnesium, and Fruit and Vegetable Intakes Are Associated with Greater Bone Mineral Density in Elderly Men and Women," American Journal of Clinical Nutrition 69 (1999): 727–36.

supermarket is unhealthy, there are a number of voices arguing that all of the harms attributed to milk do not exist with fresh milk that has not been pasteurized.

Unfortunately, it is hard to comprehensively study this question because milk is pasteurized *for a reason*: namely, to prevent the spread of infections including such potentially life-threatening illnesses, such as tuberculosis. For example, before pasteurization became prevalent, 65,000 people died from tuberculosis contracted from milk in Wales and England over a twenty-five-year span ending in 1937. Even in modern times, and with less than 1 percent of all dairy consumed in the United States being non-pasteurized, raw milk still accounted for 1,571 known cases of illness for which 202 people were hospitalized between 1993 and 2006.[16] Because of the extreme risks of serious illness or death that can be posed by raw milk, there are ethical problems with organizing studies around it. As a result, there is a dearth of solid scholarship that could clearly establish raw milk as being substantially nutritionally better than pasteurized milk.

I drank raw, unpasteurized milk from grass-grazing active cows as a kid. My grandfather kept cows, and I'd go out with him in the morning to milk them. He carefully cleaned the cow's udder, washed his hands, and used a freshly washed pail. He would carry the pail of milk straight to the wellhouse where it was surrounded by cold water. Any milk not consumed *that day* was mixed with grains and used for slopping the hogs. Exceptions occurred for my grandmother churning butter, making buttermilk, etc. (Incidentally, the milk often tasted like wild onions because the cows liked eating them!)

In that sort of situation, any microbial contamination is unlikely to be problematic, because the microbes never get an opportunity to multiply to a level that makes them any more dangerous than sticking your finger in your mouth. My grandfather also knew

---

[16] A. J. Langer *et al.*, "Nonpasteurized Dairy Products, Disease Outbreaks, and State Laws—United States, 1993–2006," *Emerging Infectious Disease* 18, no. 3 (2012).

his cows intimately. His sense of a cow's health was nothing short of amazing. So he would have noticed something like an udder infection, and he was smart about avoiding possibilities of cross-contamination that would have allowed his cows to catch sicknesses from other farms.

But my grandfather, even when I was a child, was a throwback to an earlier time. Odds are, you aren't living in circumstances even remotely similar. And those are, quite frankly, the only circumstances under which raw milk is even potentially safe to consume.

It is far more likely that you get your dairy products from a store where they are kept on a shelf anywhere from two weeks to two months (depending on the type of pasteurization used). This milk comes in handy plastic jugs delivered by a truck that picked them up from a bottling plant. The bottling plant got the milk from a gigantic tanker truck that drove two days to get there.

The cows that made the milk weren't intimately known to the people who milked them, either. Though I'm sure there are some wonderful people who work in dairies, there is a dramatic difference between the level of familiarity my grandfather had with his cows and employee number 45728 at XYZ Corporation has with cow serial numbered 314159265. Maybe that employee is incredibly conscientious, and I'm sure most agricultural employees are. But a survey of dairy employees in Wisconsin revealed serious concerns that many employees were not sufficiently literate to understand health and safety protocols, and that 30 percent of them had been injured on the job.[17]

Considering the length of time milk has to spend in supply-chain transit and in containers, combined with the very different working conditions of the modern dairy, there is simply no way that raw milk can be made safely available on a wide scale. Pasteurization is an absolute necessity for mass distribution.

Though there can be no doubt that the process of pasteurization fundamentally changes the nature of the proteins in milk—and

---

[17] P. Dyk, "Who Are Today's Dairy Employees?" *Wisconsin Agriculturist*, November 2008.

especially changes its character through the deactivation of enzymes—which means that raw milk may in fact be more healthful than pasteurized milk, I will be limiting my analysis to the stuff most people can access at their local grocery or convenience store. If you keep your own dairy cattle or goats, that's wonderful!

While on this subject, I should acknowledge that back in my grandfather's day, cows were handled differently in other ways as well. They were milked only five months out of the year and not more than a month of that was during pregnancy. Modern cows are hybridized for maximum milk production, milked for ten months a year, and kept pregnant for most of that time. This alone means modern milk has a lot more hormones than the milk of yesteryear. But we have to deal with what *is* rather than what *was* or what we'd wish!

## Milk Increases Risks of Prostate and Ovarian Cancer

Along with milk consumption increasing the risk of hip fracture in women,[18] there are also disturbing studies indicating it increases the risk of prostate cancer[19,20] in men and ovarian cancer[21] in women. A diet high in dairy also increases the risk of early menopause.[22]

Yes, you read that right. The very thing the government pushes on you as "necessary" for bone health raises your risks of early

---

[18] E. Warensjo *et al.*, "Dietary Calcium Intake and Risk of Fracture and Osteoporosis: Prospective Longitudinal Cohort Study," *BMJ* 342 (2011): d1473.

[19] M. J. Chan, *et al.*, "Dairy Products, Calcium, and Prostate Cancer Risk in the Physicians' Health Study," *American Journal of Clinical Nutrition* 74 (2001): 549–54.

[20] J. M. Chan, P. H. Gann, and E. L. Giovannucci, "Role of Diet In Prostate Cancer Development and Progression," *Journal of Clinical Oncology* 23 (2005): 8152–60.

[21] D. W. Cramer, B. L. Harlow, and W. C. Willet, "Galactose Consumption and Metabolism in Relation to the Risk of Ovarian Cancer," *Lancet* 2 (1989): 66–71.

[22] D. W. Cramer, "Epidemiologic Aspects of Early Menopause and Ovarian Cancer," *Annals of the New York Academy of Sciences*. 592 (1990): 363–75; discussion 390–94.

menopause and ovarian cancer while increasing the risks of fractures. And it isn't so good for the husband either.

Obviously, an increased risk of an undesired outcome is not the same thing as a guarantee, and people have to weigh immediate benefits (such as the need for a pint of ice cream following a nasty breakup) along with frequency of use (only once in a while, thank goodness!) against a relatively small increase in ovarian or prostate cancer risk when there's no history of it in the family. These latter risks, incidentally, are specifically tied to lactose consumption. Lactose is not present in hard cheeses.

The increased risk of bone fracture is tied more specifically to excess calcium intake and argues in favor of moderation rather than exclusion.


## Milk and Acne

Though I don't recommend deliberately sabotaging your teenager's dating life, for many teenagers a diet rich in milk yields a face full of acne. Isn't it crazy how the government pushes milk and subsidize its cost in school lunches?

Though there can be many causes of acne, the acne vulgaris prevalent in teens of both sexes and also making its appearance in many women just before their periods is caused by hormones. Hormones produced by the testicles or ovaries as well as the adrenal glands stimulate the production of cells that line sweat glands. If those cells reproduce too quickly to be cleared, the pores clog and acne results.

Every individual has a different threshold at which the total hormonal level stimulates too many cells for the sweat glands to clear. Most teens would normally remain under that threshold except for two factors: milk and stress.

Stress can stimulate an acne breakout because stress hormones generated in the adrenals add to the total level of hormones stimulating the growth of cells in the sweat glands. It is not at all uncommon for a young man or woman to experience acne for the first time in relation to a very stressful experience, such as leaving home for college or a bad breakup with a boyfriend or girlfriend. Reducing overall stress can certainly help.

But milk is also a large contributor. Milk contains hormones that add onto our normal sex hormones and adrenal hormones. In the preponderance of cases, it is the proverbial straw that breaks the camel's back and pushes a teen or young adult across the hormonal threshold into acne.

When I say "milk contains hormones," I'm not talking about the bovine growth hormones that some dairies use to stimulate milk production—though those are a problem too. Rather, I am saying that milk *naturally* contains these hormones. I don't care if the cow that made the milk spends its entire day yodeling on a pristine mountainside in the Swiss Alps and has never come into contact with human beings; its milk still contains hormones. According to the FDA, "milk cannot be produced in a way that renders it free of hormones."[23] It's that simple.

If that isn't enough to make you reconsider milk intake, milk (though not cheese) is associated with accelerated aging of the skin and wrinkles.[24]

Hormonal birth control pills can be administered that can lower the hormonal levels of girls enough that they can drink milk without causing acne eruptions, but this comes at a subtle price that can waste a lot of her time. Specifically, evidence is piling up that birth control pills alter a woman's mate preferences so that while she is on the pill, she prefers men who have major histocompatibility complex genes more similar to her own, whereas she would normally prefer men with major histocompatibility complex genes that were dissimilar.[25]

The results of willy-nilly using birth control pills, especially for such a ridiculous purpose as allowing uncontrolled consumption of milk, can be quite tragic. Researchers described matters as follows:

[23] J. Ralof, "Hormones in Your Milk," *Science News*, October 28, 2003.

[24] M. Purba *et al.*, "Skin Wrinkling: Can Food Make a Difference?" *Journal of the American College of Nutrition* 20, no. 1 (2001): 71–80.

[25] M. Wenner, "Birth Control Pills Affect Women's Taste in Men," *Scientific American*, December 2008.

*Since the Pill reverses natural preferences, a woman may feel attracted to men she wouldn't normally notice if she were not on birth control—men who have similar MHC profiles. . . .* The effects of such evolutionary novel mate choices can go well beyond the bewilderment of a wife who stops taking her contraceptive pills and notices her husband's 'newly' foul body odor. Couples experiencing difficulty conceiving a child—even after several attempts at tubal embryo transfer—share significantly more of their MHC than do couples who conceive more easily. *These couples' grief is not caused by either partner's infertility, but to an unfortunate combination of otherwise viable genes.*[26] [Emphasis added]

Most dermatologists consulted about acne issues and who recommend birth control pills as a solution are blissfully unaware of these potentially devastating side effects of birth control pills, even though the studies have been out there and repeated for at least fifteen years. Doesn't it seem crazy to take a fourteen-year-old girl, fool her body into thinking she is pregnant for years on end, and mess up her mate choices just so her body can be made compatible enough with milk that she can drink it without getting acne? Is milk really that important? Is this really a matter of health and diet—or is it some sort of strange milk-worshipping religion because of which we'll do just about anything to our kids so they can drink milk?

Let me make a more sensible recommendation that will have zero side effects: Ditch dairy *entirely*, and reduce levels of stress.

And no, I don't recommend reducing stress through putting kids on antidepressants and tranquilizers while their brains are still developing, unless it is medically indicated as a last resort. Rather, I recommend adding an exercise regimen. I'll cover exercise more comprehensively later in the book, but the link between exercise and reduced acne levels is clear. Exercise reduces levels of the stress hormone cortisol, and cortisol is one of the hormones

---

[26] F. Furlow, "The Smell of Love," *Psychology Today*, March 1996.

that cause sweat glands to clog and cause acne. The only caveat is that exercise should be followed by a shower and clean clothes.

For young men, excess adipose tissue can contribute to acne as well by altering their hormone levels. Adipose tissue tends to increase the amount of testosterone that is converted to estrogen, thereby duplicating in young men the phenomenon that young women experience near their periods. Of course, this excess adipose tissue can also cause increased social stress.

It is a good thing that I don't care if dermatologists, dairy lobbyists, grain lobbyists, and birth control pill manufacturers all hate me, because in the next paragraph I am going to summarize everything you need to know to substantively eliminate acne in nearly all cases.

The real acne solution for teens and young adults is simple: Cut out the dairy, make them step away from their social networking sites long enough to get solid exercise daily, make sure they are well acquainted with soap and water (especially immediately after exercise), and help them find ways to reduce stress. Set a bedtime that guarantees eight hours of sleep nightly as insufficient sleep raises cortisol levels. If that still doesn't work, cut out the grains. Especially for acne that persists into adulthood, a major cause is gluten sensitivity. Do all of the above for six months religiously, and the acne will be gone. Try it, and you'll see I'm right.

## Autoimmune Diseases

A certain percentage of children, if introduced to dairy too young, develop antibodies—that is an allergy—to cow's milk. Infants who develop this allergy are predisposed to develop type 1 diabetes later in childhood.[27] While not all children are at risk, because predisposition is dependent on specific genes,[28] most of us don't

---

[27] K. Luopajärvi *et al.*, "Enhanced Levels of Cow's Milk Antibodies in Infancy in Children Who Develop Type 1 Diabetes Later in Childhood," *Pediatric Diabetes* 9, no. 5 (2008): 434–41.

[28] T. Saukkonen *et al.*, "Significance of Cow's Milk Protein Antibodies as Risk Factor for Childhood IDDM: Interactions with Dietary Cow's Milk Intake and HLA-DQB1 Genotype. Childhood Diabetes in Finland Study

genetically profile our kids, so providing milk—especially at an early age—puts children at risk of needing insulin the rest of their needlessly shortened lives.

This occurs through molecular mimicry. That is, certain proteins in dairy milk resemble the surface proteins in the islet cells of the pancreas that make insulin. When the body reacts to the milk proteins and recognizes them as invaders, the antibodies generated don't just mark the milk proteins for destruction; they also mark the cells in the pancreas that make insulin. Over a period of time, those cells are silently destroyed until none are left at all. As I mentioned, this is more of a risk for people with a certain genotype—but unless you analyze your babies for this genotype to verify they can consume milk okay (and I am not aware that *anyone* has ever done this), giving your infant or toddler milk is taking a risk of also giving your bundle of joy type 1 diabetes. I realize milk mustaches are cool, but are they really worth it?

The risk of type 1 diabetes should be quite a deterrent, but as bad as that is, there are even more devastating possibilities, including multiple sclerosis. While the search for a cure for this illness continues, it is completely preventable by not giving kids milk.

Two extremely high quality studies,[29, 30] including worldwide research across population groups, have made the connection that ingestion of dairy is a prerequisite for developing multiple sclerosis later in life. Though milk ingestion alone is not enough to cause the illness, its absence is enough to prevent it.

The mechanism of causation is very similar to the way milk causes type 1 diabetes: molecular mimicry. There are proteins in milk that closely resemble the myelin oligodendrocyte glycoprotein.

---

Group," *Diabetologia* 41, no. 1 (1998): 72–78.

[29] D. Malosse *et al.*, "Correlation Between Milk and Dairy Product Consumption and Multiple Sclerosis Prevalence: A Worldwide Study," *Neuroepidemiology* 11 (1992): 304–12.

[30] D. Malosse and H. Perron, "Correlation Analysis Between Bovine Populations, Other Farm Animals, House Pets, and Multiple Sclerosis Prevalence," *Neuroepidemiology* 12 (1993): 15–27.

When the body initiates an immune response to the milk protein, the proteins of the myelin sheath get caught in the crossfire.

Though the link with Parkinson's disease is not quite as clear as with many other illnesses, a study of over 135,000 men demonstrated that milk consumption increases the risk of developing Parkinson's disease by 100 to 200 percent.[31]

Vitamin D helps to prevent autoimmune diseases by limiting the immune responses characteristic of such diseases.[32] Theoretically, the vitamin D that is required by law to be added to milk would offset the harm, but there's a problem: Calcium inhibits the absorption of vitamin D from the intestinal tract. You can bypass this problem by following your mother's wisdom: Go outside and play! The vitamin D you get from sunshine is the most potent available, and it is absorbed no matter what. Plenty of sunshine (or vitamin D supplementation—but sunshine is superior) helps to prevent the development of a wide array of autoimmune diseases.

So if you don't want your children to develop diabetes, multiple sclerosis, or Parkinson's disease, all you have to do is skip the milk and send them outside to play.

## Infections

Ear infections are a serious problem for toddlers and infants. Though the infection is usually caused by a bacterium, before an infection can take up residence, the eustachian tube needs to be blocked. In 79 percent of cases, that blockage is predisposed by a food allergen, such as milk, soy, wheat, or peanuts[33]—all things that a modern caveman should avoid feeding to kids anyway.

---

[31] H. Chen *et al.*, "Diet and Parkinson's Disease: A Potential Role of Dairy Products in Men," *Annals of Neurology* 52 (2002): 793–801.

[32] H. DeLuca and M. Cantorna, "Vitamin D: It's Role and Uses in Immunology," *FASEB Journal* 15 no. 14 (2001): 2579–85.

[33] K. Kazemka, "Could Foods Be Causing Your Child's Ear Infections?" Consumer Health Information Corporation, 2004; available at www.consumer-health.com/services/cons_take44.php.

Though I thankfully never had ear infections and neither has my daughter, the American Academy of Otolaryngology reports:

About 62 percent of children in developed countries will have their first episode of OM by the age of one, more than 80 percent by their third birthday, and nearly 100 percent will have at least one episode by age five. In the U.S. alone, this illness accounts for 25 million office visits annually with direct costs for treatment estimated at $3 billion. Health economists add that when lost wages for parents are included, the total cost of estimated treatments mount to $6 billion.[34]

Twenty-five million doctor visits and treatment cost of $6 billion! And 79 percent of that could be avoided simply by withholding foods, such as dairy, soy, and wheat, that our caveman ancestors never ate.

One piece of good news: Though it is commonly repeated as a "known fact," I've found no reliable evidence that consuming milk makes mucus either thicker or more abundant. There is one particular protein in the milk of a variety of cow that isn't typically used for milk production that may have that capacity, but the milk you buy at the store, as far as I can tell, doesn't have that effect.

## Infertility

Put down the spoon, and step away from the ice cream! While this command is not quite as important for women in their twenties, women in their mid-to late-thirties, who are already racing against time if they want to have a baby, need to pay attention.

The lactose in milk is a binary sugar composed of a molecule of glucose added to a molecule of galactose. Digestion of lactose yields galactose, which shows evidence of being toxic to ovarian

---

[34] American Academy of Otolaryngology, "Fact Sheet: Ear Infection and Vaccines"; available at www.entnet.org/HealthInformation/earInfection-Vaccines.cfm.

germ cells. The authors of this study concluded that the ability to digest lactose turned out to be a curse rather than a blessing.

> The decline in fertility with aging is steeper in populations with high per capita consumption of milk and greater ability to digest its lactose component. These demographic data add to existing evidence that dietary galactose may deleteriously affect ovarian function.[35]

Another study demonstrated that just two daily servings of low-fat dairy such as skim milk or yogurt was sufficient to increase the risk of ovulatory infertility by 85 percent.[36] And men are not immune. The more dairy a man consumes, the higher the proportion of his sperm that is abnormally shaped.[37]

If you are part of a couple having difficulty with conception, dropping dairy from your diet altogether would be a wise course.

## What About Yogurt?

I encounter advice to eat yogurt only about five times daily— on the cover of magazines, on the Internet, and in overheard conversations. There is no doubt that the live cultures in yogurt (and buttermilk) can be a worthy addition to one's intestinal flora. Unfortunately, they come at a price.

The first is that the lactose in yogurt hasn't been completely converted to lactic acid. As a result, all of the detriments of lactose (such as infertility problems) apply. Further, in manufacturing yogurt, it isn't heated to high enough temperatures to denature

---

[35] Daniel W. Cramer, Huijuan Xu, and Timo Sahi, "Milk Products and Ovarian Function Adult Hypolactasia, Milk Consumption, and Age-Specific Fertility," *American Journal of Epidemiology* 139, no.3 (1994).

[36] J. E. Chavarro, *et al.*, "A Prospective Study of Dairy Foods Intake and Anovulatory Infertility," *Human Reproduction* 22, no. 5 (2007): 1340–47.

[37] M. Afeiche *et al.*, "Dairy Food Intake in Relation to Semen Quality and Reproductive Hormone Levels Among Physically Active Young Men," *Human Reproduction* 28, no. 8 (2013): 2265–75.

the proteins and hormones. Thus, all of the risks that pertain to milk also apply to yogurt.

In addition, you may notice that the advice is to consume *unsweetened* yogurt. Yet, when I looked for unsweetened yogurt at the supermarket, out of eighty shelf-feet, only about six inches was dedicated to one container of one brand of unsweetened yogurt. The conclusion is obvious: People prefer and choose to consume sweetened yogurt. I looked at the nutritional label on a popular brand of yogurt, and then I looked at the label on Coca Cola. It turns out that, ounce for ounce, this popular brand of "healthy" yogurt contains more sugar than the leading sugared soft drink.

Sugar is sugar. Your body is going to respond to it identically no matter what sort of label is applied to it. It makes zero sense to consume something with more sugar than a soft drink and consider it healthy.

But, it is even worse than that. Milk all by itself or in products, such as yogurt or cottage cheese, raises insulin levels far higher than the sugar or lactose present in the product would predict. This is particularly the case with the low-fat and skim products most often recommended.[38] Because of this phenomenon, consumption of low-fat milk and yogurt has a distinct tendency to stall attempts at weight loss. Whether sweetened or not, the reason for this is the unique mix of amino acids present in milk. This mix of amino acids was designed by nature to make calves gain weight quickly, and it works well on humans too.

The benefits to intestinal flora are actually a very important matter, but there are some aspects to this that are important to consider. Specifically, if you are eating a diet rich in fruits and vegetables while excluding grains, legumes, and dairy, you will not be doing a great deal of bovine-style fermentation in your gut. Provided you don't get dosed with antibiotics, you will consume plenty

---

[38] C. Hoppe *at al.*, "High Intakes of Milk, but not Meat, Increase S-Insulin and Insulin Resistance in 8-Year-Old Boys," *European Journal of Clinical Nutrition* 59 (2005): 393–98.

of bacteria on the surface of the food you eat, which benefits your intestinal flora.

## What About Aged and Hard Cheeses?

Aged and hard cheeses have excluded or converted practically all lactose, so they don't present problems with fertility if consumed. The specific amino acids that tend to spike insulin when dairy is consumed are contained in the whey, and whey is excluded from hard cheeses. So hard cheese won't create the same insulin spike as even unsweetened yogurt.

Beyond this, cheese presents a mixed picture. On the one hand, it still contains hormones that can increase risks of prostate and ovarian cancers as well as contribute to acne in teens and young adults. The proteins it contains can trigger autoimmune reactions, especially in infants and toddlers, that can lead to development of insulin-dependent diabetes and multiple sclerosis.

In addition, cheese is perhaps one of the most calorie dense foods in existence, meaning that you shouldn't eat gobs of it if you are trying to lose weight. But it can be hard for some people to cut down on cheese, because the casein protein in cheese is far more concentrated than the casein in milk, and casein releases casomorphin—an opioid peptide—when it hits the stomach. And yes, the effects can include tolerance—which is the medical term for addiction.[39]

On the other hand, as we'll examine in a later chapter, the government, nutritional, and medical communities hold some fundamentally flawed beliefs regarding fats. Cheese is high in saturated fats. Though conventional wisdom dictates that saturated fat is evil and will put you in an early grave from heart disease, actual studies on the specific effects of cheese, butter, and full-fat dairy indicate that they substantially *reduce* the risk of heart

---

[39] W. Hurley and M. Aslam, "Biological Activities of Peptides Derived from Milk Proteins," *Illini DairyNet*, University of Illinois Extension, August 5, 1998.

disease.[40] The dairy fat is high in natural vitamin D, vitamin K2, vitamin E, and vitamin A. It is also rich in valuable medium-chain triglycerides, omega-3 fatty acids, and butyric acid—all of which are good for you. Consistently for decades, consumption of full-fat dairy products has been linked with lower risks of stroke and lower risks of heart disease overall.[41]

Even better, the more dairy fat one consumes, the lower the person's risk of developing insulin resistance or type 2 diabetes.[42]

## Summary Recommendations on Dairy

Don't give milk or yogurt to infants or toddlers. Don't consume any dairy products if you are having trouble with acne. Don't consume milk, yogurt, cottage cheese, kefir, or similar products if you are female and have concerns about ovulatory infertility—especially if you have delayed childbearing past age thirty.

Butter, hard cheeses, and aged cheeses raise the risk of prostate and ovarian cancer but lower the risk of heart disease, stroke, and type 2 diabetes. Depending on your own family history of these diseases, you can choose to either avoid them *or* consume them in moderation. Moderation means you will eat them no more than three times a week because of their extreme caloric density and addictive potential.

Eat butter as a condiment whenever it's appropriate or the mood strikes if you have no acne issues.

---

[40] M. Bonthius *at al.*, "Dairy Consumption and Patterns of Mortality of Australian Adults," *European Journal of Clinical Nutrition* 64 (2010): 569–77.

[41] P. Elwood *et al.*, "Milk Consumption, Stroke, and Heart Attack Risk: Evidence from the Caerphilly Cohort of Older Men," *Journal of Epidemiology and Community Health* 59, no. 6 (2005): 502–5.

[42] M. Healy, "Dairy Component Shows Promise in Cutting Diabetes Risk," *Los Angeles Times*, December 20, 2010.

# Chapter 6
# Myths, Realities, and What You Need to Know About Fats

A war was started on fat (especially saturated and animal fats) and cholesterol in the United States in the late 1960s and was officially incorporated into the dietary recommendations of government agencies and the medical establishment in the early 1970s.

We were told that this war would result in better cardiovascular health, lower rates of cancer, lower rates of obesity, and lower rates of diabetes. As animal fats and saturated fats in our diet were replaced with vegetable oils, hydrogenated vegetable oils, and high glycemic carbohydrates in a bid to make us healthier, we have instead become more ill. In practically every measure of health, we have become substantially less healthy.

So let's stand back and take a look at the results Americans have experienced from the first major dietary guidelines in the 1970s through the various modifications of those guidelines until today. If the recommendations of the USDA and various heart-health and cancer-prevention organizations are at all effective, we should have seen major decreases in death rates since then. Since the 1970s, fast-food restaurants have replaced lard with canola oil for frying, popcorn vendors at movie theaters have abolished coconut oil from their products, processed food manufacturers have done everything possible to exclude fat, and practically everything you can buy has so-called heart-healthy versions and is "rich in antioxidants."

Given all of this—the consciousness raising of Americans and even the responsiveness of fast food enterprises, combined with medical advances—we should see a serious improvement in the health of Americans over the past forty years. That is, *if* the dietary recommendations are *valid*, we should see amazing improvement.

The USDA started its war on fat in 1970 by specifying that our diet should consist of four servings of bread, pasta, and grain;

four servings of fruits and vegetables; three servings of dairy; and two servings of meat and fish daily. By the time the USDA food pyramid was developed in 1992, the USDA was recommending at least six but no more than eleven servings daily from the "bread, cereal, rice, and pasta" group, and just two or three servings daily from the "meat, poultry, fish, dry beans, eggs, and nuts" group. In other words, according to the USDA, an ideal diet could exclude meat altogether so long as you added some black beans to your plate full of spaghetti.

So how have these USDA guidelines that waged a war on calories from animal fat and meat so they could be replaced with calories from starches and "healthy" vegetable oils worked out for Americans? Poorly.

According to the National Institutes of Health, in 1970 fewer than 15 percent of adult Americans were obese, but by 2009 that number had hit 35.7 percent.

Since 1970, smoking prevalence among adults has dropped from 40 to 20 percent. As smoking is the single most pervasive preventable cause of cancer, you'd logically expect our death rates from cancer to have declined precipitously. According to the mortality maps generated by the National Cancer Institute website, between 1970 and 1974, 1,719,792 people died from cancer out of a population of 209,896,021. Between 2000 and 2004, 2,772,461 people died from cancer out of a population of 281,421,906.[1]

So in the early 1970s, 205 out of every 100,000 people died from cancer annually. In the early 2000s, the annual rate of cancer deaths was 20 percent higher: 246 per 100,000.

How can that be, you ask? I'm sure you've seen numerous news reports about the progress being made on cancer treatment. Even the National Cancer Institute reports a decline in death rates. Why are my numbers inconsistent?

The numbers I am giving you are *raw*. They are just facts. X people out of a population of Y died from cancer. The news articles

---

[1] Cancer statistics are provided by the National Cancer Institute. Population statistics are estimates from the U.S. Census Bureau.

you see generally pertain to cures for relatively rare forms of cancer, and the decline in deaths reported by the National Cancer Institute is based on an arbitrary age adjustment. That is, since the population of the United States is aging, they subtract out the cancer deaths of people they think might have died from other causes anyway. Really. But the cold, hard reality is in the numbers I have reported without any arbitrariness or fudge factors, and of course they include medical advances in early detection and treatment of cancers.

According to data published by the Centers for Disease Control,[2] the incidence of diagnosed diabetes in the United States amounted to 1.62 percent of adults in 1968. By 2008, that number had more than tripled—and nearly quadrupled—to 6.29 percent. According to the American Heart Association, the prevalence of high blood pressure has also increased.[3]

In 1980, the U.S. population was approximately 226,546,000, of whom approximately 640,000 had a major inpatient cardiac procedure annually.[4] This is 282 procedures per 100,000 people per year. In 2005, the U.S. population was approximately 295,108,000, of whom approximately 2,640,000 had a major inpatient cardiac procedure. This is 894 procedures per 100,000 people annually. Cardiac procedures tripled in only twenty-five years.

I've just thrown a lot of numbers at you, for which I apologize. But I believe if I'm going to tell you something that flies in the face of conventional wisdom, I should substantiate it. If your eyes glazed over, let me summarize: In spite of the fact that the percentage of people smoking has been cut in half since 1970, and in

---

[2] Centers for Disease Control, "Long Term Trends in Diagnosed Diabetes," October 2011; available at www.cdc.gov/diabetes/statistics/slides/long_term_trends.pdf.

[3] American Heart Association, "Heart Disease and Stroke Statistics 2012 Statistical Update"; available at http://my.americanheart.org/professional/General/Heart-Stroke-2012-Statistical-Update_UCM_434526_Article.jsp.

[4] Data from American Heart Association, "Heart Disease and Stroke Statistics 2012 Statistical Update," U.S. Census Bureau, *National Vital Statistics Report* 60, no. 3, *Monthly Vital Statistics Report* 23, no. 8.

concert with official recommendations emphasizing a grain-based diet and replacing animal fats with vegetable oils, the prevalence of cancer, heart disease, high blood pressure, obesity, and diabetes have increased. In some cases they have doubled or tripled.

Albert Einstein is famously quoted as defining insanity to be "doing the same thing over and over again and expecting different results." We are getting *horrible results,* and it is high time we subjected the recommendations we are being given to serious scrutiny rather than doubling down on approaches that have a forty-year proven track record of actually worsening the problems they purport to solve.

The results speak for themselves in stark and indisputable terms. The only question is whether or not we are willing to resolve the cognitive dissonance between what we believe and what is real by modifying our beliefs to match reality or by ignoring what is real and adopting ever more tortured arguments to explain away increasingly disparate results.

We've already gone over "healthy" grains and legumes, so let's move on to "horrible" fats.

## Types of Fat

The words used to describe dietary fats can be confusing. This is mainly because the words are based in chemistry and thrown around by journalism and communications majors who are quite frankly unfamiliar with chemistry but extremely familiar with political advocacy. So they use the words describing dietary fats with inflections reminiscent of words like "harlot" or "abomination." A second factor adding to the confusion is that, in spite of what marketing people and other propagandists put forth, very few naturally occurring fats are homogeneously of one type. Most natural fats contain a mixture of various sorts of fat.

Most journalists will describe lard as containing saturated fat, olive oil as being a monounsaturated fat, and canola oil as containing polyunsaturated fat. This is an extreme oversimplification. The olive oil in my cabinet, for example, contains 10 g of monounsaturated fat, 2 g of polyunsaturated fat, and 2 g of saturated fat per serving; the lard in my refrigerator contains 5.7 g of saturated fat, 6.1 g of monounsaturated fat, and 1.3 g of polyunsaturated fat per serving; and a jug of safflower oil at the grocery store (*not* in my cabinet for reasons I'll explain) has 11 g of polyunsaturated fat, 1 g of saturated fat, and 2 g of monounsaturated fat per serving.

In reading many authors, I find that they usually justify skipping an explanation of the mechanics of fats on the grounds that the audience will find it boring. What I say is this: Provide the information and let the reader decide what is interesting. Unless you work for the mafia or CIA, there's no such thing as knowing too much. Also, the more you know, the more readily you can detect misinformation.

There are three types of naturally occurring dietary fats: saturated, monounsaturated, and polyunsaturated.

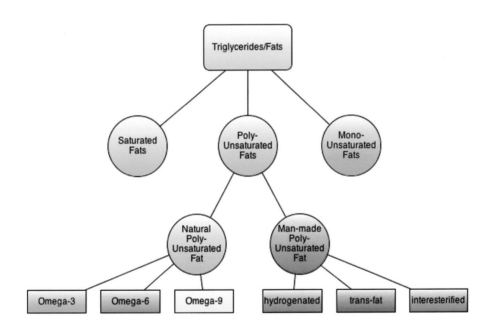

All fats are triglycerides. A glyceride is an ester formed by combining glycerol (an alcohol) with any of a number of fatty acids. Esters are made by practically any combination of an acid and an alcohol. Glycerides are a special case in which the alcohol involved is always glycerol, also known as glycerin. So glycerin combines with a fatty acid to make a glyceride. Three glycerides combine to make a triglyceride—also known as fat.

Fatty acids consist of a hydrocarbon chain terminated with a COOH group. It is this terminating COOH group that makes it an acid rather than a hydrocarbon that you'd put into your fuel tank. In fact, the manufacture of biodiesel from vegetable oils is accomplished by removing this group along with the glycerol from the oil—leaving the hydrocarbon.

Each carbon in a chain has four bonds available. In a saturated fatty acid, each carbon is bonded to two hydrogen atoms and two adjacent carbon atoms (except for the first carbon in the chain, which is combined with three hydrogens and the second carbon). This sort of fatty acid is called saturated because it can hold no more hydrogen atoms in its structure.

Fat is said to be unsaturated when two adjacent carbon atoms share a double bond, thus leaving room for two more hydrogen atoms (or atoms of some other element). This unsaturated state makes unsaturated fats less stable and more reactive, meaning that they will oxidize or become rancid more easily.

Unsaturated fats are either monounsaturated—meaning there is only one double bond in the chain—or they are polyunsaturated, meaning that there is more than one double bond.

There are many varieties of saturated, monounsaturated, and polyunsaturated fatty acids. Most that occur naturally have between four and twenty-eight carbons, and the number of carbons is an even number. If you have ever read the ingredients on a bottle of shampoo, the names of some of these fatty acids, such as oleic, stearic, and palmitic acids, will sound familiar.

The hydrogen atoms in a polyunsaturated fatty acid can be arranged in either a "cis" configuration or a "trans" configuration. Most naturally occurring unsaturated fatty acids have a "cis" arrangement, meaning that the hydrogen atoms are on the same side of the double bond. With the notable exception of vaccenic acid, which occurs naturally in beef and dairy, fatty acids with a "trans" arrangement, in which the hydrogen atoms are on opposite sides of the double bond, are a result of industrial processes.

The industrial process that creates trans fats is called *hydrogenation.* It is accomplished by combining a vegetable oil containing a lot of polyunsaturated fatty acids with hydrogen gas under tremendous heat and pressure. The end result is a form of fat that does not exist at all in nature and is insanely dangerous. Whereas the single type of trans fat found in beef and dairy actually *reduces* the risk of heart disease,[5, 6, 7] man-made trans fats are recognized to present extraordinary risks to cardiovascular health. A study review in the *New England Journal of Medicine* summarized the matter nicely as follows: "On a per-calorie basis, trans fats appear to increase the risk of CHD more than any other macronutrient, conferring a substantially increased risk at low levels of consumption (1 to 3 percent of total energy intake)."[8] Hydrogenated vegetable oils in all forms should be avoided.

The data pertaining to trans fat was so compelling that many government bodies sought to ban or regulate it. In response, the manufacturing industry has switched to interesterified fats. Referring to the explanation of triglycerides, the process of interesterification involves mixing different fats together and then using catalysts or enzymes to switch which fatty acids are connected to which glycerol in the molecules. There has not yet been an exhaustive body of research on these fats, so I cannot say with certainty if they are harmful or not. What I *can* say is that these fats, like trans fats, are novel to the human body and produced by an industrial process. So it is pretty certain we aren't well adapted to them.

---

[5] "Alberta Natural *Trans* Fat Research Earns Global Recognition," International Symposium on Chylomicrons in Disease (ISCD) report, April 2008; available at www.meristem.com/meeting/iscd_2008-02.htm.

[6] "Trans Fats From Ruminant Animals May Be Beneficial—Health News," *redOrbit*, September 8, 2011; available at www.redorbit.com/news/health/2608879/trans-fats-from-ruminant-animals-may-be-beneficial/.

[7] C. M. C. Bassett *et al.*, "Dietary Vaccenic Acid Has Antiatherogenic Effects in LDLr-/- Mice," *Journal of Nutrition* 140, no. 1 (2010): 18–24.

[8] D. Mozaffarian *et al.*, "Trans Fatty Acids and Cardiovascular Disease," *New England Journal of Medicine* 354, no. 15 (2006): 1601–13.

Looking more closely at unsaturated fats, there are three types of unsaturated fat that play a notable role in our health—particularly as it pertains to their ratio. These are called omega-3, omega-6, and omega-9 fats. The name and number comes from which carbon in the chain holds the double bond that makes the fat unsaturated. If it is the third carbon in the chain, then it is omega-3; if it is the sixth carbon in the chain, then it is omega-6.

Another category of fat worth mentioning involves the conjugated fatty acids. Conjugated fatty acids are polyunsaturated fatty acids in which two double bonds are separated by just one single bond. The most notable dietary example is conjugated linoleic acid (CLA). CLA is present primarily in the meat and milk of ruminants, but it is also present in kangaroos and can be synthesized in the gut by intestinal bacteria. CLA tends to change body composition in favor of lean muscle mass and has notable anti-inflammatory properties.

## The Role of Fats in the Body

When it comes to natural dietary fats, there is no such thing as "good" or "bad" per se. All of these fats play an important role in the optimal function of our bodies. What makes a particular fat "good" or "bad" is more a matter of quantity (specifically, the ratio of that fat in our diet in comparison with other fats) and how it is used.

The specific fatty acids in saturated fats are important for cellular communication, and about half of the material in our cell membranes is saturated fat. Saturated fat is necessary for immune function and calcium uptake, and is used in synthesizing other necessary fats in the body. Because it is saturated, it is very chemically stable. As such, it is ideal for frying foods because it can withstand high heats without becoming oxidized into compounds that put oxidative stress on the body. I'll explain why this is important later.

Saturated fat can raise your overall cholesterol, but interestingly enough, it does so in a way that is beneficial. Specifically, saturated fat lowers the proportion of the most damaging types of cholesterol (LDL-B and HDL-3) in your blood. Though it has long been accepted with theological certitude that saturated fat increases your risk of heart disease, this is not true.

Remember from the last chapter on dairy foods that researchers have discovered that, despite the high amount of saturated fat in dairy products, those who consumed the most dairy fat had the lowest risks of heart disease? The most comprehensive meta-analysis to date covering over 300,000 people and examining the results of studies in which saturated fat intake was correlated to actual heart disease, stroke, or cardiovascular disease concluded that there is *absolutely no relationship* in either direction.[9]

Monounsaturated fats are present in lard, tallow, olive oil, sunflower oil, avocados, and many other sources, though they are best known for their presence in olive oil.

The primary monounsaturated fatty acid present in olive oil is oleic acid, though oleic acid also makes up 44 percent of the fatty acid content of lard and is the most prevalent fatty acid in human fat. Oleic acid has been demonstrated to play a critical role in immune function.[10] There is evidence that diets high in monounsaturated fat are cardio-protective.[11, 12]

Until relatively recently, the primary use for industrially processed polyunsaturated fats was in paints and varnishes. In fact, I have a bookcase in my bedroom that I finished with linseed (also known as flax) oil. Polyunsaturated fats are chemically reactive and prone to oxidation, which makes them an excellent choice for

---

[9] P. W. Siri-Tarino *et al.*, Q "Meta-Analysis of Prospective Cohort Studies Evaluating the Association of Saturated Fat with Cardiovascular Disease," *American Journal of Clinical Nutrition* 91, no. 3 (2010): 535–46.

[10] C. Carrillo, M. Cavia Mdel, and S. Alonso-Torre, "Role of Oleic Acid in Immune System; Mechanism of Action; a Review," *Nutricion Hospitalaria* 27, no. 4 (July–August, 2012): 978–90.

[11] F. B. Hu *at al.*, "Dietary Fat Intake and the Risk of Coronary Heart Disease in Women," *New England Journal of Medicine* 337 (1997): 1491–99.

[12] S. M. Artaud-Wild *et al.*, "Differences in Coronary Mortality Can Be Explained by Differences in Cholesterol and Saturated Fat Intakes in 40 Countries but not in France and Finland: A Paradox," *Circulation* 88 (1993): 2771–79.

varnishing furniture and a very poor choice for cooking or frying, as they become a source of free radicals, carcinogens, and oxidative stress on the body.[13] Polyunsaturated fats start to turn into trans fats when heated to temperatures as low as 120°F. This is why replacing saturated fats with polyunsaturated fats has been demonstrated to increase the risk of death from all causes, including cardiovascular disease.[14]

Within the general category of polyunsaturated fat, there are a couple of special cases: omega-6 and omega-3 fats. The human body needs both types of fat for fueling various processes, but it is best adapted to consuming these fats in a ratio of omega-6 to omega-3 of between 4:1 and 1:1—the lower the better.[15] We achieved this naturally when most of the fat we ate came from small sea creatures and wild game.

The primary omega-6 oil in the human diet is linolenic acid (LA) and the primary omega-3 oil in the diet is alpha linolenic acid (ALA). The body processes ALA into eicosapentaenoic acid (EPA) and then converts the EPA to docosahexaenoic acid (DHA). It is this latter compound—DHA—that is probably the most powerful naturally occurring anti-inflammatory compound on earth. The human body is not very efficient at converting ALA to EPA and ultimately into DHA in the first place, but what figuratively and literally drives the nail into the coffin is the fact that when omega-6 is consumed in excess, it tends to monopolize the metabolic pathways that allow the body to create DHA. Thus, consuming an excess of omega-6 relative to omega-3 compromises the body's innate ability to fight

---

[13] V. Scislowski *et al.*, "Effect of Dietary N-6 and N-3 Polyunsaturated Fatty Acids on Peroxidizability of Lipoproteins in Steers," *Lipids* 40, no. 12 (2005): 1245–56.

[14] C. Ramsden *et al.*, "Use of Dietary Linoleic Acid for Secondary Prevention of Coronary Heart Disease and Death: Evaluation of Recovered Data from the Sydney Diet Heart Study and Updated Meta-Analysis," *BMJ Group.*

[15] P. A. Simopoulos, "The Importance of the Ratio of Omega-6/Omega-3 Essential Fatty Acids," *Biomedicine & Pharmacotherapy* 56, no. 8 (2002): 365–79.

inflammation, leading to higher risks of heart disease and cancer.[16, 17]

The most widely used vegetable oils are soybean and corn oil, whose ratios of omega-6 to omega-3 are 7.7:1 and 46:1, respectively.

Keeping in mind that the human body doesn't convert ALA into EPA/DHA very well (and that our ability to make the conversion is compromised both by aging and by excess consumption of omega-6), it is not enough that ALA be consumed. We are better off, in fact, including both EPA and DHA directly in our diet. Vegetable oils, including canola oil and flaxseed oil, when they include omega-3s, contain ALA only and no EPA or DHA. When animal fats contain omega-3s, a majority of those omega-3s are in the form of EPA and DHA, which can be used directly by our bodies without need for inefficient conversion.

The human brain contains substantial amounts of DHA (and cholesterol, incidentally), and there is solid evidence that the expansion of brain size noted in modern and early modern humans was facilitated by our consumption of animal foods high in DHA—most notably seafood.[18, 19] The National Institutes of Health recommend that pregnant women consume at least 300 mg of DHA daily and that children under age three consume at least 150 mg daily. In practice, most pregnant women consume less than 80 mg daily.[20] About

---

[16] A. Park, "Omega-6 Fats Linked to Increased Risk of Heart Disease," *Time*, February 6, 2013; available at http://healthland.time.com/2013/02/06/omega-6-fats-linked-to-increased-risk-of-heart-disease/.

[17] M. Hughes-Fulford *et al.*, "Arachidonic Acid Activates Phosphatidylinositol 3-Kinase Signaling and Induces Gene Expression in Prostate Cancer," Cancer Research 66, no. 3 (2006): 1427–33.

[18] C. L. Broadhurst *et al.*, "Brain-Specific Lipids from Marine, Lacustrine, or Terrestrial Food Resources: Potential Impact on Early African Homo Sapien,"*Comparative Biochemistry and Physiology Part B: Biochemistry and Molecular Biology* 131 (2002): 653–73.

[19] S. C. Cunnane and M. A. Crawford, "Survival of the Fattest: Fat Babies Were the Key to Evolution of the Large Human Brain," *Comparative Biochemistry and Physiology Part A: Molecular & Integrative Physiology* 136 (2003): 17–26.

[20] NIH Workshop (Bethesda, MD, 1999).

96,000 U.S. deaths annually can be *directly* attributed to insufficient DHA intake.[21]

Domesticated poultry has an omega-6 to omega-3 ratio of 9:1, as opposed to 2:1 for wild poultry, and the amount of EPA/DHA present in grain-fed cattle is only one-tenth of that present in wild cattle. Both venison and bison are very high in EPA/DHA[22] as well. Wild elk and deer have an omega-6 to omega-3 ratio of 2:1, as do grass-fed steers. Grain-fed steers, however, are more likely to have a ratio of 13:1.[23]

In practice, most people simply do not have access to free-ranging chickens, grass-fed beef, or venison they hunted. If such food is available at all, it is available at exorbitant prices. This means seafood is the way to get these crucial fatty acids into the diet. However, two cautions are in order: Because of high mercury content, the larger fish such as tuna, shark, and swordfish should be eaten no more than once a week (and avoided altogether during pregnancy), and there is a substantial difference between wild and farm-raised fish. In many cases, farm-raised fish are effectively useless.[24]

The omega-6 to omega-3 ratio of the fat in a given food doesn't tell the whole story. Though I see a lot of websites where those ratios are listed, they don't take into account the fact that polyunsaturated fats such as these are, in many cases, a small amount of the total fat. Beef fat from conventionally raised beef, for example, contains 52 percent saturated fat, 44 percent monounsaturated fat, and only 4 percent polyunsaturated fat. So if you eat a tablespoon of pure beef fat, you'll get 500 mg of polyunsaturated fat,

---

[21] *PLoS Medicine* 6, no. 4 (2009).

[22] M. Crawford *et al.*, "Fatty Acid Ratios in Free Living and Domestic Animals, in Modern Dietary Fat Intakes in Disease Promotion," *Nutrition and Health* (2010): 95–108.

[23] B. Watkins, "Experts Offer the Skinny on Search for Healthy Fat," *Purdue News*, February 4, 2002.

[24] B. Holub, "Omega-3 Levels in Fish: Data Quality, Quantity and Future," 2009 National Forum on Contaminants in Fish, Portland, OR, November 4, 2009; available at http://water.epa.gov/scitech/swguidance/fishshellfish/fishadvisories/upload/day3f.pdf.

of which 450 mg are omega-6 and 50 mg is omega-3. If you are aiming for a 1:1 ratio, all you have to do is eat a can of sardines (containing 1,000 mg of omega-3) to balance out two tablespoons of pure beef fat from the worst industrial feedlot operation.

But vegetable oils are another matter. Soybean oil (used ubiquitously in salad dressings), for example, is 60 percent polyunsaturated fat, and a tablespoon of soybean oil will give you a whopping 7,000 mg of omega-6s balanced by only 900 mg of omega-3s. You'd have to eat six cans of sardines to balance out the inflammation effects of just one tablespoon of soybean oil! Overall, you are much better off eating a portion of steak trimmed of external fat, especially given that numerous studies show steak (and meat generally) to have an overall beneficial effect on blood lipids.[25, 26]

## Are Industrial Vegetable Oils Food?

There's no doubt that many people consume vegetable oils as though they were food, but it is important to ask if this is a good idea. The example given regarding soybean oil above also applies to corn oil and many others. The only widely available vegetable oils that don't present the problem of insane levels of omega-6 fats are flax, walnut, canola, sunflower, coconut, palm, and olive oil.

Olive oil, flax oil, walnut oil, sunflower oil, palm oil, and coconut oil can all be derived from their sources using primitive equipment without need of solvents, hydraulic pressure, or heat. When these come out of the press, they are accompanied by natural antioxidants and vitamins.

Olive oil is predominantly a monounsaturated fat, and coconut oil is predominantly a saturated fat, so these two fats are pretty

---

[25] M. A. Denke, "Role of Beef and Beef Tallow, an Enriched Source of Stearic Acid, in a Cholesterol-Lowering Diet," *American Journal of Clinical Nutrition* 60 (1994): 1044S–49S.

[26] E. Beauchesne-Rondeau *et al.*, "Plasma Lipids and Lipoproteins in Hypercholesterolemic Men Fed a Lipid-Lowering Diet Containing Lean Beef, Lean Fish, or Poultry," *American Journal of Clinical Nutrition* 77, no. 3 (2003): 587–93.

stable. The coconut oil in particular is good for frying and cooking, because its stability allows for use at higher temperatures (up to about 350°F) without creating toxic byproducts. Olive oil (when it hasn't been fraudulently mixed with some other oil—which is very common[27]) is healthful. Both of these are clearly food.

But if you were to press your own flax or walnut oil, you'd find that it goes bad at room temperature in short order because the high proportion of polyunsaturated acids makes them easily oxidized—so you'd have to store them in the refrigerator. You'll recall my mentioning earlier that I finished furniture with linseed (flax) oil. Just boiling it and then exposing it to air turns it into varnish. But if properly stored, these are healthy and worthy of the designation of being "food" as well.

In fact, all of the oils that can be produced using primitive equipment and without reliance on solvents, hydraulics, or high temperatures are healthful. In essence, these are the oils that would have been available to a caveman. One thing to keep in mind, however, is that despite their favorable omega-6 to omega-3 ratio, nearly all of their omega-3 is present as ALA, and your body will only convert about 1 percent of it to needed DHA[28]—and that assumes a best-case scenario. In order to get the necessary 300 mg of DHA needed daily from flax seed oil, for example, you'd need to eat enough of it to get 30,000 mg of ALA—or about five tablespoons, which is a bit over a quarter of a cup. But before you get excited, I suggest you try some flax oil. Most people I know find it utterly unpalatable. When I make salad dressings using olive oil, I'll use about 20 percent flax or walnut oil in place of some of the olive oil, and then it's okay.

I didn't mention canola oil above, and there's a good reason. Though it is advertised as having a favorable 2:1 ratio of omega-6 to omega-3 fats, those polyunsaturated fats go through a heavy-duty industrial process that includes deodorizing at high temperatures,

---

[27] T. Mueller, *Extra Virginity: The Sublime and Scandalous World of Olive Oil* (New York: W. W. Norton & Company: 2013).

[28] B. Anderson and David W. L. Ma, "Are All N-3 Polyunsaturated Fatty Acids Created Equal?" *Lipids in Health and Disease* 8 (2009): 33.

extraction with chemical solvents, and pressing at high temperatures. In other words, it is an industrial product. Polyunsaturated fats will naturally go rancid in short order if kept at room temperature, yet you can open a bottle of canola oil and then leave it at room temperature for weeks without apparent change. Do you refrigerate your canola oil—or any of your vegetable oils for that matter? I don't know anyone who does.

So why don't they go bad? The first reason is because of trans fats. As you'll recall, man-made trans fats are so nasty they shouldn't be eaten at all, but manufacturers convert vegetable oils into trans fats so their products have longer shelf lives. The process of making canola oil for table use converts as much as 4 percent (2 percent on average) of it into trans fats.[29] So why isn't that fact on the label? Because the serving size of oil is 13 g; anything less than 0.5 g of trans fats is allowed by law to be reported as "zero," and 2 percent of 13 g is 260 mg. So you get 260 mg of this poison in every tablespoon of canola oil, and *it doesn't even appear on the label.*

It's even worse in restaurants. Have you ever gone into a restaurant where they proudly advertise that all of their frying is done in "heart-healthy canola oil?" The canola oil used for deep fryers is not the same product you buy in the grocery store. To lower its "smoke point," it is hydrogenated, and the end result contains a whopping 21 percent chemically manufactured trans fat![30]

The second reason for the room-temperature stability of industrially made polyunsaturated oils is their extreme purity. When you are synthesizing something in the laboratory, purity is good. For example, all trace minerals (especially of a metallic nature) are removed from industrial vegetable oils. This is because their presence hastens rancidity and makes them less stable. With oils that

---

[29] Sean. O'keefe, Sara. Gaskins-Wright, Virginia. Wiley, I-Chen. Chen, "Levels of Trans Geometrical Isomers of Essential Fatty Acids in Some Unhydrogenated U. S. Vegetable Oils," *Journal of Food Lipids* 1, no. 3 (1994): 165–76.

[30] "Oil, Vegetable, Industrial, Canola (Partially Hydrogenated) Oil for Deep Fat Frying," SELF*NutritionData*; available at http://nutritiondata.self. com/facts/fats-and-oils/7948/2; accessed on June 27, 2013.

are mostly monounsaturated (such as olive oil) or saturated (such as coconut oil), they don't need to be removed. As a result, these latter oils contain a host of beneficial nutrients and vitamins. But industrial vegetable oils are 100 percent chemically pure. It's like the difference between having a glass of wine—which contains resveratrol and other antioxidants along with calcium, magnesium, choline, and potassium—and the chemically pure ethyl alcohol used as an industrial solvent. Wine is food, but Sterno™ isn't.

Chemically pure substances are great for making pharmaceuticals, paints, dyes, plastics, and a wide array of useful products, but they are not *food*.

## The Bottom Line on Fats

All forms of artificially created fats should be avoided because they are effectively deadly poisons. Just 2 percent of your daily caloric intake coming from trans fats will double your risk of heart disease. Anything that is hydrogenated, interesterified, processed under tremendous heat and pressure, extracted with petroleum solvents, or otherwise treated like an industrial product is precisely that: an industrial product. It is absolutely positively *not* food, and you consume it at your peril. Soybean and corn oil have so much omega-6 fatty acid content that eating them promotes a plethora of chronic diseases, so they should be avoided like the plague.

Naturally occurring vegetable fats that can be derived through cold-pressing are perfectly fine. This includes walnut oil, flax oil, coconut oil, palm oil, and olive oil among others. Though oils such as walnut oil and flax oil have beneficial omega-6 to omega-3 ratios, only 1 percent of the omega-3 that they contain can be converted into something useful in the body. So vegetable oils high in polyunsaturated fatty acids should be used in caveman moderation. Vegetable oils that are high in polyunsaturated fat should be refrigerated and should never be used for cooking.

Natural (i.e., cold-pressed and not chemically purified) vegetable oils high in monounsaturated fat, such as olive oil and avocado oil, tend to be cardioprotective. Though there is no limitation on their use, it should be kept in mind that they have a lot of calories. (A tablespoon of oil has 126 calories.) Both olive oil and avocado oil can be used for cooking and frying at temperatures up to 375–400°F.

Natural vegetable oils high in saturated fat, such as coconut and palm kernel oils, are safe to eat and popular for cooking. The smoke point of coconut oil is just a bit higher than 350°F, so it should be kept below that temperature. Palm kernel oil is one of the most stable cooking oils of vegetable origin, with a smoke point of 450°F. With both of these, it is worth getting the "virgin" (meaning cold-pressed) product because otherwise you get something that has been refined into an industrial product. Saturated fats do tend to raise cholesterol, and they are high in calories, so you shouldn't eat them by the pound just for fun. But their effect on cholesterol is beneficial overall in that they lower the proportions of the most dangerous (LDL-B and HDL-3) types of cholesterol.

The fats from animals have a healthy effect overall, though the omega-6 to omega-3 ratio of animals raised in commercial operations tends to be bad. But because the amount of their polyunsaturated fat is small, the contribution they make to inflammation can be easily countered by trimming visible fat and including seafood in the diet. Fats from wild animals obtained by hunting or from grass-fed and free-ranging animals are extremely beneficial. The omega-3 fats they contain are predominantly in forms such as EPA and DHA that can be used directly by the body to immediately counter inflammation.

Dairy fat has been demonstrated repeatedly to lower the risk of cardiovascular disease. It is high in CLA, which shows promise in reducing inflammation generally[31] and fighting cancer.[32, 33]

---

[31] J. Bassaganya-Riera, R. Hontecillas, and D. C. Beitz, "Colonic Anti-inflammatory Mechanisms of Conjugated Linoleic Acid," *Clinical Nutrition* 21, no. 6 (2002): 451–59.

[32] X. Y. Ke *et al.*, "The Therapeutic Efficacy of Conjugated Linoleic Acid-Paclitaxel on Glioma in the Rat," *Biomaterials* 31, no. 22 (2010): 5855–64.

[33] J. I. Jung *et al.*, "Trans-10,cis-12 Conjugated Linoleic Acid Inhibits Insulin-Like Growth Factor-I Receptor Signaling in TSU-Pr1 Human Bladder Cancer Cells," *Journal of Medicinal Food* 13, no. 1 (2010): 13–19.

This has to be balanced with the risks of dairy outlined in the previous chapter. For young children, dairy should be avoided to prevent type 1 diabetes and multiple sclerosis. In teens, it can cause acne. In general, especially with warehoused cattle, its high hormone levels (which are much higher than the hormone levels in our grandparents' milk) can increase the risk of hormone-sensitive cancers of the breast and prostate while impairing fertility of both men and women. On the other hand, hard or aged cheeses in particular have a lot of beneficial fat that can help prevent cardiovascular problems and reduce inflammation. How you choose to handle that depends on your other risk factors.

Like wild animals, seafood contains a lot of omega-3 fat. Because so much of the fat is in the form of DHA, it should be considered a dietary necessity at least three times a week. Wild seafood is best because many farm-raised fish are nutritionally useless. A CNN article regarding farm-raised salmon stated, "Nearly all salmon Americans eat are farm-raised—grown in dense-packed pens near ocean shores, fed fish meal that can be polluted with toxic PCB chemicals, awash in excrement flushed out to sea, and infused with antibiotics to combat unsanitary conditions."[34]

Larger species of fish, such as swordfish and shark, tend to concentrate toxic metals like mercury, so they should be eaten only once a week and avoided by pregnant women. Smaller species, such as salmon, sardines, herring, and anchovies contain tons of DHA. When choosing tuna, the "white albacore" contains about three times as much DHA as "light" or "chunk light" tuna. It is fine to eat these canned (packed in water—not oil), and this is usually the least expensive way.

At the fish counter, wild salmon tends to be quite expensive. Here are some less expensive options that contain a lot of DHA: wild arctic char, wild Atlantic mackerel, black cod (aka sablefish), oysters, mussels, and halibut. At my local grocery store, you can

---

[34] M. Jampolis, "Is Farm-Raised Salmon as Healthy as Wild?" *CNN Health*, January 8, 2010; available at www.cnn.com/2010/HEALTH/expert.q.a/01/08/salmon.fresh.farmed.jampolis/.

buy many varieties of wild-caught fish in prefrozen bags for about $6/lb. If you like to go fishing, many freshwater species are high in EPA/DHA as well, including bass, whitefish, catfish, lake herring, and lake trout.

Eggs are likewise a good source of EPA/DHA. These are contained in the yolk, and two egg yolks will provide 304 mg of EPA/DHA. Keep in mind, though, that omega-3 fats are polyunsaturated, so to preserve the benefits, you shouldn't overcook them. If frying, keep the yolk runny; otherwise, boil them to make a soft- or hard-boiled egg. Eggs are much maligned because they contain cholesterol, but the advice to limit egg intake is outdated. Numerous studies now show that even eating more than three eggs daily has a net beneficial effect on blood lipids.[35] Though American organizations have been slow to change their recommendations, the British Heart Foundation has already updated its recommendations to include eggs as part of a healthy diet.

So, eat your steak and eggs, enjoy some fish, and use some olive oil. In other words, eating the fats our caveman ancestors ate is perfectly healthy. Avoid fats that require an industrial civilization to produce.

## Let's Talk About Cholesterol

Cholesterol is a core building block of the body and it is mainly produced in the liver. Cholesterol is used by the body for practically everything—to make our sex hormones, make vitamin D from sunshine, heal wounds, make digestive enzymes, and more. It is a core component of the myelin sheath of our neurons. Dietary cholesterol (like you'd get from eating eggs or shrimp) is not absorbed directly into the bloodstream and is, in fact, broken down in the intestines. The reason it isn't absorbed directly into

---

[35] C. M. Greene, *Response to Dietary Cholesterol and Carotenoids Provided by Eggs, in an Elderly Population*, 2006 doctoral dissertation; available at http://digitalcommons.uconn.edu/dissertations/AAI3223344.

the bloodstream is because cholesterol is insoluble in water, blood, or other bodily fluids.

When the liver makes cholesterol, it encapsulates the cholesterol in a protein that allows the blood to carry it to where it is needed. When the capsule reaches its destination, the cholesterol is dropped off, and the protein gets recycled. The core of the capsule—the cholesterol—is the same in all cases, and it is a perfectly safe and necessary part of our bodies. In fact, it is so essential that many people on cholesterol-lowering medication experience horrendous side effects, including severe memory loss.[36]

The capsule is what makes the difference. The liver will put the cholesterol into capsules of different types and sizes depending on a number of factors, including how much sleep you are getting, how much stress you are under, what your state of inflammation is, and most importantly, what kind of food you eat. Though it is currently fashionable to divide cholesterol into two forms: HDL (high-density lipoprotein), or "good" cholesterol, and LDL (low-sensity lipoprotein), or "bad" cholesterol, that is a vast oversimplification at best and deceptive at worst.

Though it is true that both HDL and LDL exist, in terms of your health these designations are meaningless. There are at least three types of HDL and at least three types of LDL. The thing that makes the difference between these various types of HDL and LDL—and makes those types more or less dangerous—is their *size*. When it comes to the capsules surrounding cholesterol, size matters.

The smaller something is, the more reactive it is. That is, the more easily it combines with other substances. Probably one of the most dramatic examples of this idea is wheat. All by themselves, wheat kernels will burn with difficulty if you give them plenty of oxygen. But if you mill the kernels of wheat into a fine dust (also known as flour), it becomes a devastating explosive when suspended in air. (Think of the many fatal grain elevator explosions.) The particles of cholesterol are like that. Larger particles of either

---

[36] D. Graveline, *Lipitor Thief of Memory: Statin Drugs and the Misguided War on Cholesterol* (Haverford, PA: Infinity, 2006).

HDL or LDL tend to be mild mannered and even protective, but the small particles are highly reactive, which makes them more dangerous.

Though some forms of both HDL and LDL are smaller and thus more reactive than others, none of them are in and of themselves dangerous until they meet with one of four processes: oxidation, inflammation, glycation, or stress. You can consider these four things to be the four horsemen of your body's apocalypse.

Oxidation is, to some degree, a natural process. Our cells naturally produce unpaired electrons (known as free radicals) to facilitate metabolism. In an ideal situation, these free radicals are kept in check by the antioxidants we consume and generate within our bodies, so the damage they can do is limited. Vitamin C is perhaps the best-known antioxidant, but there are dozens of others we consume naturally in fruits and vegetables. Our body also makes antioxidants, including coenzyme Q10. Coenzyme Q10 is made in the liver along the same metabolic pathway that makes cholesterol. Guess what statin drugs lower along with cholesterol? Yep—coenzyme Q10. So if you are taking a statin drug, at a bare minimum you need to be taking a coenzyme Q10 supplement.

With a diet rich in fruits and vegetables, our bodies can handle the levels of oxidation inherent in normal body processes. But in the modern world, we also do things that increase the number of free radicals in our bodies such as inhale ozone in a polluted city, engage in extended exercise, smoke, or eat polyunsaturated fats that have been used for frying. Particularly if our diet has insufficient fruits and vegetables, these activities will generate free radicals that aren't kept in check and can pair with—and damage—other molecules in our bodies, including cholesterol. It is here that the smaller and more reactive cholesterol particles become dangerous because these are the ones damaged by free radical oxidation, and when they are damaged, they will cause arterial and heart diseases.

I bet you were surprised to see "extended exercise" mentioned right next to smoking in the previous paragraph. I first started to suspect this when I learned that Jim Fixx, the author of *The*

*Running Book* and a hero of mine when I ran track, had died quite young from a heart attack. Over the years, evidence has mounted that extended exercise, due to which the body is in a constant state of inflammation and there isn't sufficient rest to allow antioxidants to neutralize the free radicals, can have the same net effect as heavy smoking in terms of oxidative stress. Exercise confers enormous health benefits and helps to prevent practically all chronic diseases—up to the equivalent of thirty total miles of running weekly. But when you go beyond that, the body can't recover adequately, and you wind up achieving the opposite.[37] Studies show that overdoing exercise (meaning the equivalent of more than thirty miles of running weekly) also correlates to cognitive decline in women.[38]

The smaller a particle of cholesterol of either HDL or LDL happens to be, the more reactive it is, and thus the more easily it is oxidized. The relative proportions of these smaller particles is definitely important and—unlike measurements of total cholesterol, LDL cholesterol, or HDL cholesterol—is predictive of heart disease. Unfortunately, this is not something doctors usually test. Triglycerides are also predictive of heart disease, most especially the ratio of triglycerides to HDL cholesterol. And all of these factors are indeed affected by diet—though not in the way the dominant dietary theology would predict.

One of the reasons (but not the only one as we'll soon see) why replacing saturated fats, such as animal fat and coconut oil, with vegetable oils, such as soybean and corn oil, leads to increased heart disease is that vegetable oils are high in polyunsaturated fats. Polyunsaturated fats are less stable when subjected to the high heat of cooking or frying and quickly mutate into compounds that are carcinogenic and place oxidative stress on the body. Though it may have been expedient given the propaganda campaign waged against them, when fast-food outlets went to polyunsaturated vegetable oils for frying, they weren't doing us any favors.

---

[37] K. Helliker, "The Exercise Equivalent of a Cheeseburger? New Research Says Endurance Running May Damage Health," *Wall Street Journal*, May 24, 2013.

[38] J. Barron, "Strenuous Exercise Makes Jane Dumb," 2009; available at www.jonbarron.org/article/strenuous-exercise-makes-jane-dumb.

Inflammation is also a problem. In this respect, I am not speaking so much about acute inflammation (such as occurs with a cut that is healing) as with the chronic and body-wide inflammation that goes unnoticed for month after month and year after year while it increases our risk of practically every disease of civilization. Inflammation is the absolute key factor in heart disease[39] as well as cancer.[40] Heart disease starts with inflammation, and it is inflammation that initiates the cascade of events that culminates in a heart attack.

One thing that will cause inflammation is eating foods to which your body has an immune response. As discussed in previous chapters, nearly a third of people have measurable immune responses to gluten, but given the lectins and molecular mimicry exhibited by grains, legumes, and (to a lesser extent) dairy, the elimination of at least the first two items and the severe restriction of the latter to only hard or aged cheeses and butter in moderation will go a long way toward preventing heart disease.

The other major cause of inflammation is our high carbohydrate diet. More than perhaps any other factor, the advanced glycation end (AGEs) products created by a diet in which carbohydrates provide most of the calories are a nightmare. I'll delve into the mechanism in greater depth in the next chapter, but the high blood sugar a carbohydrate-based diet creates causes glucose in the blood to combine with proteins—including the proteins encapsulating cholesterol. Proteins are normally slippery, but the glycation makes them sticky, and these proteins damage the inner walls of our arteries and vessels. When they become damaged and inflamed, the liver sends help in the form of healing cholesterol, but our heavy omega-6 intake combined with a high carbohydrate diet means that most of the cholesterol sent is encapsulated in the small reactive particles that easily oxidize, glycate, and become sticky.

---

[39] J. Bowden and S. Sinatra, *The Great Cholesterol Myth: Why Lowering Your Cholesterol Won't Prevent Heart Disease—and the Statin-Free Plan That Will* (Beverly, MA: Fair Winds Press, 2012).

[40] D. Agus, *The End of Illness* (New York: Free Press, 2012).

Here again, our industrial vegetable oil diet comes to the fore. Normally, our bodies could cope with the temporary assault of a bit of chocolate cake, but as we explored in the previous section, vegetable oils tend to be extremely high in omega-6 polyunsaturated fats, and what little omega-3 polyunsaturated fat they contain is in a form the body can barely use. Because of this, they shut down our body's natural checks and balances on inflammation so it can rage out of control. In addition, this imbalance causes our cells to crank out inflammatory cytokines. This cycle of inflammation is only checked by a radical change of diet or fatal illness.

Another factor adding to inflammation is being overweight. When you have too many fat cells in your body—likely caused by our carbohydrate-heavy diet as I'll explain in the next chapter—those cells constantly emit inflammatory substances that contribute to practically all causes of death other than misadventure.[41]

Oxidation, glycation, and inflammation are all exaggerated by stress. Stress revs up your body's production of the more reactive forms of cholesterol,[42, 43] causes insulin resistance,[44] raises blood sugar,[45] and increases inflammation throughout the body.[46]

---

[41] T. E. Brinkley et al., "Total and Abdominal Adiposity Are Associated with Inflammation in Older Adults Using a Factor Analysis Approach," *Journals of Gerontology Series A: Biological Sciences and Medical Sciences* 67, no. 10 (2012): 1099–106.

[42] C. Catalina–Romero et al., "The Relationship Between Job Stress and Dyslipidemia," *Scandinavian Journal of Public Health* 41, no. 2 (2013): 142–49.

[43] A. Steptoe and L. Brydon, "Associations Between Acute Lipid Stress Responses and Fasting Lipid Levels 3 Years Later," *Health Psychology* 24, no. 6.

[44] L. S. Brandi et al., "Insulin Resistance of Stress: Sites and Mechanisms," *Clinical Science* (London) 85, no. 5 (1993): 525–35.

[45] R. Wing et al., "Psychologic Stress and Blood Glucose Levels in Nondiabetic Subjects," *Psychosomatic Medicine* 47, no. 6 (1985).

[46] Duke Medicine News and Communications, "Anger, Hostility and Depressive Ssymptoms Linked to High C-Reactive Protein Levels," *DukeHealth. org*, September 22, 2004; available at www.dukehealth.org/health_library/news/8164.

So cholesterol itself is not a problem. Fats normally found in nature are not a problem. The real problem is the high carbohydrate diet promulgated by a misguided government and health sector combined with the promotion of industrially produced oils that are dramatically more dangerous than even the fat of warehoused cattle. When our government started pushing whole grains and vegetable oils as an antidote to heart disease, it was like sending a gas tanker to put out a fire. It has been a disaster for millions of Americans who died before their time. There has to be a better way.

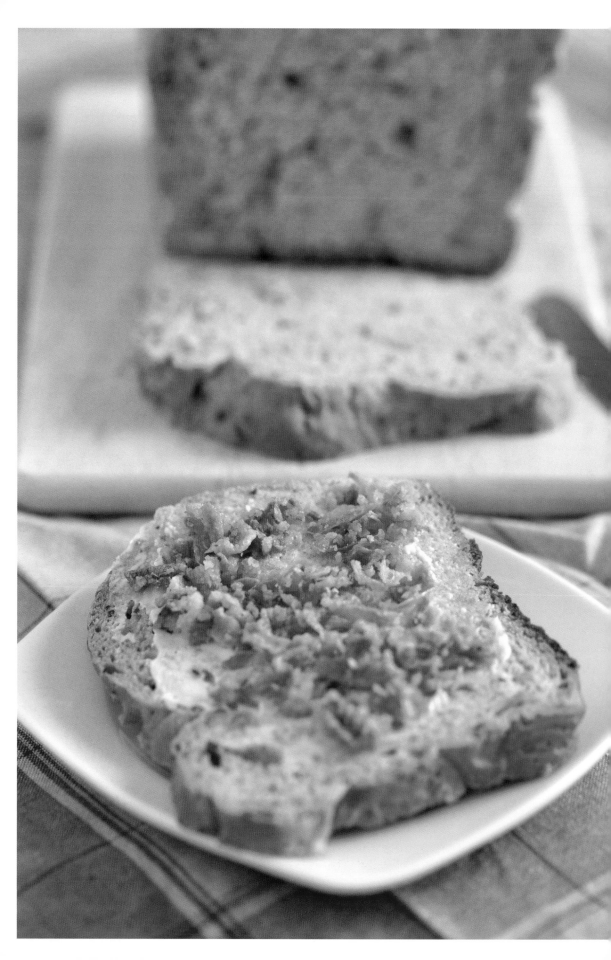

# Chapter 7
# Carbohydrates: Dangerous Curves Ahead

For decades there was a sign along Interstate 95 in Providence, RI, advertising an adult club. It stated plainly "Dangerous Curves Ahead." If you've ever been along that stretch of road, you know the sign served a dual purpose because the road wends its way around dangerous curves, left-hand merges, and more. It's a very dangerous road, just like the carbohydrate-based diet urged upon us by government agencies and far too many health professionals who should know better. They should know better because the research is abundant and clear on this topic.

There is no doubt that our bodies evolved with an ability to digest many forms of carbohydrates. From the ptyalin in saliva to the amylase in the small intestine, the body has a well-evolved ability to digest and assimilate carbohydrates. Though it is extremely common for people to have adverse reactions to milk, gluten, or beans—it is practically unheard of for someone to have an adverse reaction to broccoli or carrots. Though I have heard people espouse a diet containing no carbohydrates whatsoever, in light of our broad evolutionary adaptation to them, the idea seems ludicrous.

There is no question that we should be consuming natural highly complex carbohydrates such as cabbage, onions, and other fruits and vegetables. In fact, vegetable consumption alone increases lifespan and decreases the risk of practically all chronic diseases.[1] A couple of years ago I wrote a book about vegetable gardening,[2] and I found through research that the sheer vitamin content, antioxidant

---

[1] C. Li *et al.*, "Serum -Carotene Concentrations and Risk of Death Among U.S. Adults: The Third National Health and Nutrition Examination Survey Follow-up Study," *Archives of Internal Medicine* 171, no. 6 (2011): 507–15.

[2] B. Markham, *Mini Farming Guide to Vegetable Gardening: Self-Sufficiency from Asparagus to Zucchini* (New York: Skyhorse Publishing, 2011).

content, and other beneficial effects of vegetables are striking. The benefits are so extreme that even the World Health Organization classifies some vegetables, such as onions, as medicine.[3]

So the question of whether or not carbohydrates should be eaten is a closed case: of course you should eat them.

But, when most people think of carbohydrates, they aren't thinking about the carbohydrates that our caveman ancestors ate, such as the progenitors of our modern pears, kale, peaches, and onions. Rather, we think of mashed potatoes, whole-grain cereal, bread, crackers, cake, and candy bars. But there is a world of difference between a bowl of whole-grain cereal and an apple.

You've already read the chapter on why you shouldn't eat grains. I think I documented the case against grain well enough to convince practically any skeptic, but pretend for a moment that you skipped that chapter or simply don't believe the volumes of evidence. Even if you skip the issues of antinutrients, lectins, and gluten, the whole-grain cereal, bread, crackers, and mashed potatoes are bad for you for another reason: they are practically devoid of nutrients (except those that were artificially added), and they are concentrated pure sugar.

Let's compare a stalk of broccoli to a bowl of the popular whole-grain cereal Grape Nuts™. I'm using this brand of cereal as an example because it was my favorite back when I ate grains. I'd fill up a bowl, slice a banana on top, put some rice milk on it, and have a side of peanut butter toast. Yummy!

First off, let's be honest about the serving size. The serving size is stated as "1/2 cup," and anyone knows that when you eat cereal, you fill the bowl, and then float it in milk. So you really eat at least a full cup. Have you ever carefully measured half a cup of cereal into a bowl? I guess it's possible that you have, but so far I've never seen anybody do it. But let's be generous and assume people really use measuring cups with their cereal. A half-cup serving of this cereal contains 37 g of nonfiber carbohydrate.

---

[3] World Health Organization, *WHO Monographs on Selected Medicinal Plants*, vol. 1 (1999); available at http://apps.who.int/medicinedocs/en/d/Js2200e/3.html#Js2200e.3.

A foot-long stalk of broccoli (weighing about a pound) contains 11 g of nonfiber carbohydrate.

The stalk of broccoli has almost twice as much dietary fiber as the cereal, 303 percent of the RDA of vitamin C, 87 percent of the RDA of vitamin A, and a bunch of cancer-fighting antioxidants, and it has a glycemic load of 8. (I'll have more to say about glycemic load shortly.) The broccoli contains vitamins and antioxidants that will protect your cholesterol from oxidation, and the glycemic load is so low that glycation is a nonissue.

On the other hand, the cereal has no vitamin C, it has 21 percent vitamin A, and although it has 123 percent of the RDA for iron, that iron was actually added (check the ingredients) as iron oxide. Iron oxide is a polite name for *rust*. It's the exact same rust as on the rusty pliers mountain men use to pull teeth rotted from eating cereal. I have no idea if the body absorbs rust as a nutrient as well as it would absorb iron from spinach or steak, but let's just assume you were intended to eat rust and its good for you. On the other hand, the cereal has a glycemic load of 28.

How can a cereal with practically no sugar have such a high glycemic load? The answer is because dietary carbohydrates are just long strands of sugar, and once they hit the small intestine, digestive enzymes break them down into glucose in short order. Even if you are eating a biscuit that contains no sugar at all, when it gets to your small intestine, every bit of carbohydrate in that biscuit turns into pure sugar. At that point, your body reacts no differently to a biscuit than it would to a few tablespoons of sugar. This is the danger of a high-carbohydrate diet. Our bodies evolved to handle a bit of sugar in an apple or to break down the carbohydrates in vegetables, but they were never intended to cope with 2,000 calories a day in carbohydrates that turn into pure sugar shortly after being eaten.

## Glycemic Load and Why It Matters

Perhaps if you are diabetic or know someone who is diabetic, you've heard of glycemic index. The glycemic index of a food is a measure of how quickly it raises blood sugar when compared with pure glucose or white bread. Though this number is interesting, it doesn't mean much by itself because it doesn't take the quantity of food consumed into account. The number that takes both glycemic index and quantity into account is called glycemic load. This gives a general idea of not only how quickly it will raise blood sugar but also for how long the blood sugar will be elevated. So every food has a particular glycemic load based upon its constitution and quantity.

The human body regulates blood sugar within a very narrow range through the hormones insulin and glucagon. When blood sugar is too high, insulin is released to force glucose into the cells. When blood sugar is too low, glucagon is released to bring that glucose back out of the cells into the bloodstream. Insulin is such an important hormone that it is present in all animals, even fish.[4]

Glucose is the fuel for all of our cells, and our cells store glucose that isn't immediately needed in the form of glycogen. The glycogen in our cells becomes depleted during exercise, and as the cells start requiring more glucose, the glycogen stores in the liver are converted into glucose by glucagon. This is why if you are going to eat something with a high glycemic load, it is best to do so shortly following strenuous exercise. At that time, the store of glycogen in your muscles is depleted so that when your blood sugar rises from eating, the insulin response will push the sugar into your muscle cells to restore your supply of glycogen.

But what happens if your blood sugar rises, insulin kicks in, and your cells already have plenty of glycogen because you haven't been exercising? Well, that glucose has to go somewhere. While the glucose level is elevated, it causes glycation of proteins leading to arterial damage and worse. To minimize the damage, the body puts it in the only place it can: fat cells.

As long as our fat cells are responsive to insulin, we can theoretically gorge ourselves on candy all day, and the only side effect is we'll get fatter and fatter. Of course, we'd be suffering from the

---

[4] M. A. Caruso and M. A. Sheridan, "New Insights into the Signaling System and Function of Insulin in Fish," *General and Comparative Endocrinology* 173, no. 2 (2011): 227–47.

effects of glycation while the excess glucose gets shuttled into our fat cells. And those fat cells will increase our bodies' levels of generalized inflammation. This is why being more than just a few pounds overweight can dramatically decrease life span. But that's not the worst of it. High carbohydrate diets raise the risk of developing insulin resistance, metabolic syndrome, and more.[5]

This is where glycemic load comes into play. A caveman diet doesn't allow for consumption of concentrated sugars, such as fruit juice, processed sugar, or grains as a concentrated source of carbs. In fact, the only time substantively concentrated carbs, such as potatoes, are consumed is closely following vigorous exercise—when glycemic load is a nonissue. A caveman diet has an extremely low total glycemic load. That is what humans are best adapted for.

When we go against our evolution and eat a high glycemic load diet, the damage to our health in practically every respect is incalculable. A high glycemic diet creates advanced glycation end products that damage our blood vessels by making them more permeable,[6] accelerate the aging of capillaries,[7] disrupt the chemistry of the delicate endothelium in blood vessels,[8] enhance inflammation,[9] and keep blood vessels from dilating properly.[10]

---

[5] C. E. Finley *Et al.*, "Glycemic Index, Glycemic Load, and Prevalence of the Metabolic Syndrome in the Cooper Center Longitudinal Study," *Journal of the American Dietetic Association* 110, no. 12 (2010): 1820–29.

[6] E. Svensjo *et al.*, "Vascular Permeability Increase as Induced by Histamine or Bradykinin Is Enhanced by Advanced Glycation Endproducts (AGE)," *Journal of Diabetes and its Complications* 13 (1999): 187–90.

[7] S. Yamada and C. Ohkubo, "The Influence of Frequent and Excessive Intake of Glucose on Microvascular Aging in Healthy Mice," *Microcirculation* 6 (1999): 55–62.

[8] K. Otero *et al.*, "Albumin-Derived Advanced Glycation End-Products Trigger the Disruption of the Vascular Endothelial Cadherin Complex in Cultured Human and Murine Endothelial Cells," *Biochemical Journal* 359 (2001): 567–74.

[9] G. Basta *et al.*, "Advanced Glycation End Products Activate Endothelium Through Signal-Transduction Receptor RAGE: A Mechanism for Amplification of Inflammatory Responses," *Circulation* 105 (2002): 816–22.

[10] G. Rashid *et al.*, "Effect of Advanced Glycation End-Products on Gene Expression and Synthesis of TNF-Alpha and Endothelial Nitric Oxide Synthase by Endothelial Cells," *Kidney International* 66 (2004): 1099–106.

A meta-analysis incorporating over 400,000 study participants concluded, "High dietary glycemic load is associated with a higher risk of CHD and stroke, and there is a linear dose-response relationship between glycemic load and CHD risk."[11] In plain English, this means that the more "healthy whole grains" and sugar you eat, the more likely you are to get coronary heart disease or have a stroke.

Glycemic load is also associated with the risk of recurrence of colon cancer, and the increased insulin production required by high glycemic diets is a factor in tumor growth and recurrence for cancers generally.[12] High glycemic load also increases the risk of age-related macular degeneration. I could bore you with citations of dozens of studies, but instead I will summarize: High carbohydrate intake and the resulting high glycemic load dramatically increase the risk of everything from going blind or having erectile dysfunction to getting diabetes, heart disease, and many cancers.

At the beginning of the chapter on fats, I went down a list of all the problems our government-approved diet was supposed to solve and how every one of those problems has gotten worse instead of better. Along with industrial fats, a major contributor to that phenomenon is the central role of carbohydrates in our diet.

One aspect of health that is often a cause for concern is declining fertility. It turns out that high carbohydrate intake leads to lower sperm count in men[13] and increases the risk of ovulatory infertility in women.[14]

---

[11] J. Fan *et al.*, "Dietary Glycemic Index, Glycemic Load, and Risk of Coronary Heart Disease, Stroke, and Stroke Mortality: A Systematic Review with Meta-Analysis," *PLoS ONE* 7, no. 12 (2012).

[12] J. A. Meyerhardt *et al.*, "Dietary Glycemic Load and Cancer Recurrence and Survival in Patients with Stage III Colon Cancer: Findings from CALGB 89803," *Journal of the National Cancer Institute* 104, no. 22 (2012): 1702–11.

[13] J. E. Chavarro *et al.*, "Carbohydrate Intake and Semen Quality Among Young Men," *ASRM annual meeting*, 2012.

[14] J. E. Chavarro *et al.*, "A Prospective Study of Dietary Carbohydrate Quantity and Quality in Relation to Risk of Ovulatory Infertility," *European Journal of Clinical Nutrition* 63, no. 1 (2009): 78–86.

## Carbohydrates and Aging

There is no magic bullet to cure aging. Eventually, we'll all get old, and if we live long enough and avoid all other diseases, we will eventually die from something.[15] This is simply the nature of being born a mammal. Perhaps, eventually, this riddle will be solved, but for now I regret to say I have no magic cure for aging.

But what I can tell you is that getting a handle on carbohydrates will substantially improve your odds of living a longer life and getting the most out of life at every age. It all goes back to insulin. The more your diet forces your body to depend on insulin, the greater the damage. But that damage doesn't just take place outside your cells—it takes place inside them as well, especially with your mitochondria.

Mitochondria look like small bacteria inside your cells. This resemblance may not be entirely coincidental, as it is theorized that the mitochondria in our cells arose from a symbiosis with a proteobacteria.[16] Mitochondria have their own DNA that is separate from that contained in the chromosomes of the nucleus. Though they are involved in many cellular processes, their most well known role is producing most of the energy required by the cell.

The DNA contained in the chromosomes in the cell nucleus comes with a lot of safeguards against faulty replication and damage[17], whereas mitochondrial DNA has only one mechanism to protect itself from being damaged by free radicals: the antioxidant superoxide dismutase. High carbohydrate diets create a cellular environment in which superoxide dismutase is insufficient to

---

[15] D. Agus, *The End of Illness* (New York: Free Press, 2012).

[16] J. Reece *et al.*, *Campbell Biology.* 9th ed. (San Francisco: Benjamin Cummings, 2010).

[17] B. Alberts *et al.*, *Molecular Biology of the Cell*, 4th ed. (New York: Garland Science, 2002).

prevent damage to mitochondrial DNA from free radicals.[18, 19] This leads to injury to the mitochondrial DNA.[20] Because there are few mechanisms for correcting this damage, the damage accumulates with each division of the cell.

Though this is certainly not the only mechanism involved in aging, it is a major mechanism, and most importantly, it is something within our power to control.

## Wrinkled Old Prune?

We've all seen people who look radiant and beautiful in late middle age and people in their mid thirties who look like they have one foot in the grave and another on a banana peel. Though part of this difference is genetic, lifestyle has a lot to do with it. The three most important factors over which you have control are alcohol consumption, carbohydrate consumption, and eating enough vegetables.

Alcohol damages your skin in myriad ways. It dilates capillaries near the skin's surface more than they would usually dilate. This isn't a problem if it happens once in a while, but if it happens habitually, the capillaries become damaged, leading to the blotchiness seen in the skin of many alcoholics. In addition, the toxic aspects of alcohol have been demonstrated to cause premature aging (where the effects of age occur earlier than expected) and exaggerated aging (where the effects of age occur more severely than expected).[21]

---

[18] S. Gregersen *et al.*, "Inflammatory and Oxidative Stress Responses to High-Carbohydrate and High-Fat Meals in Healthy Humans," *Journal of Nutrition and Metabolism* 2012, article ID 238056 (2012).

[19] I. Slesak, W. Haldas, and H. Slezak, "Influence of Exogenous Carbohydrates on Superoxide Dismutase Activity in *Trifolium repens* L. Explants Cultured In Vitro," *Acta Biologica Cracoviensia, Series Botanica* 48, no. 1 (2006): 93–98.

[20] K. F. Petersen and G. I. Shulman, "Etiology of Insulin Resistance," *American Journal of Medicine* 119, no. 5, suppl. 1 (2006): S10–S16. Review.

[21] R.L. Spencer and K.E. Hutchison, "Alcohol, Aging, and the Stress Response," *Alcohol Research & Health* 23, no. 4 (1999).

The body can handle and detoxify a certain amount of alcohol without adverse effects, but it is when this threshold is exceeded that damage accumulates, leading to premature aging of every cell in the body, including skin. How much is too much? Science currently says that moderate drinking may be beneficial but that anything exceeding that is bad. How is "moderate" defined? It is defined as *one drink* or *less* for women and *two drinks* or *less* for men no more than twice weekly. How much is in a drink? Five ounces of wine, twelve ounces of beer, or one and a half ounces of distilled 80-proof liquor constitute one drink. It is important for women in particular to understand that the female body is not equipped to handle alcohol as well as man's. It isn't just because of size—the liver enzymes work differently. If a man and a woman are the same size and drink the same amount of alcohol, it will affect the woman more severely. That's why the limits for men and women are different.[22]

If you want to look your best at any age, a key factor in avoiding wrinkles and having radiant skin is restriction of high glycemic carbohydrates. The damage done by sugars on mitochondrial DNA applies to every cell and system in the body: brain tissue, heart tissue and even your skin. Along with damage to mtDNA in skin cells, elevated blood sugar causes skin damage by glycating the collagen that keeps skin supple and wrinkle free. When the collagen becomes glycated, it becomes stiff and damaged.[23, 24]

Eating fruits and vegetables is the third easily controlled factor in skin aging. Studies show that no matter where someone lives or whether he or she smokes, a diet high in green leafy vegetables,

---

[22] National Institute on Alcohol Abuse and Alcoholism, "Women"; available at www.niaaa.nih.gov/alcohol-health/special-populations-co-occurring-disorders/women.

[23] N. Perricone, *The Perricone Prescription: A Physician's 28-Day Program for Total Body and Face Rejuvenation* (New York: William Morrow Paperbacks, 2004).

[24] J. F. Vliegenhart and F. Casset, "Novel Forms of Protein Glycosylation [Review]," *Current Opinion in Structural Biology* 8 (1998): 565–67.

fructose combined with 50 percent glucose.) The small amounts of fructose naturally present in fruits is not a problem, because the amount is small and it is more than offset by the other benefits provided by the fruit. But when eaten in large quantities without any compensating benefits, it is extremely dangerous.

Fructose cannot be used directly by cells and is handled by the liver. Fructose intake (including from table sugar, corn syrup, and high fructose corn syrup) leads to the production of smaller cholesterol packets, and these smaller cholesterol packets are more easily oxidized and dramatically more dangerous than they would otherwise be. (Please see Chapter 6 for more on this.) The level of triglycerides in the blood is increased. To make matters worse, even though fructose provides sweetness and calories, unlike glucose it doesn't suppress the release of ghrelin—one of the major hormones stimulating appetite.

So when you eat something sweetened with fructose, you literally have to eat twice as much of it to get the same sensation of fullness as you'd get from eating something sweetened with glucose. Meanwhile, the liver is busy cranking out fats left and right while altering your cholesterol profile for the worse.

In sum, grains, table sugar, corn syrup, and high fructose corn syrup are not safe. What is?

Obviously, overindulgence in any carbohydrate can be problematic, but you can eat up to 70 g of a safe carb (or a combination of safe carbs) following vigorous exercise. Which ones are safe?

Honey. Honey doesn't raise your blood sugar as quickly as either table sugar or glucose,[28] and it contains a mix of twenty-four different sugars.[29] It does contain fructose, so it should definitely be used in moderation (meaning no more than three times a week), but it also contains a host of other beneficial substances to offset its fructose content if used moderately in connection with exercise.

---

[28] P. Shambaugh, V. Worthington, and J. H. Herbert, "Differential Effects of Honey, Sucrose, and Fructose on Blood Sugar Levels," *Journal of Manipulative and Physiological Therapeutics* 13, no. 6 (1990): 322–25.

[29] P. Stanway, *The Miracle of Honey: Practical Tips for Health, Home and Beauty* (London: Watkins Publishing, 2013).

It is important not to heat honey higher than 104°F to retain its beneficial enzymes.

Root vegetables. Root vegetables, including (but not limited to) parsnips, sweet potatoes, and potatoes are safe to use moderately in connection with exercise, assuming you don't have a specific allergy or adverse reaction to them. A single potato provides 63 g of carbs, and a cup of parsnips has 17 g.

White rice. Although rice is a grain, when the bran is removed all of the lectins and antinutrients go with it. White rice is as close to a pure carbohydrate as you are likely to find. A cup of cooked white rice has 45 g of carbohydrate.

Fresh and dried fruits combine simple sugars with important nutrients.

These ingredients could be creatively mixed into a sort of "recovery dessert." For example, cooked white rice could be mixed with raisins and a bit of honey to make a rice pudding.

Keep portion size in mind. The figure of 70 g of carbohydrates I gave above is for someone who has run so far that he or she has "hit the wall" and has no glycogen reserves left. Most ordinary exercise falls short of that, so you might only need 40 g or 50 g. This isn't something you need to measure with a scale. Instead, just be honest with yourself. Does picking up the TV remote control qualify as vigorous exercise? Is doing 10 push-ups comparable to running a marathon? Are your legs shaking from glycogen depletion?

## The Bottom Line on Carbohydrates

You should aim to get your carbohydrates from fruits and vegetables. You should avoid concentrated sugars, such as fruit juice, jams, jellies, table sugar, and corn syrup. You should certainly avoid grains and legumes as a source of carbohydrates. Fructose should be avoided outside of its natural context within a fruit or vegetable.

If you are a very active person, your body is designed to accommodate more concentrated carbohydrates during a two-hour window following intense exercise. You can replenish your glycogen during this time with fruits, but it may be easier to use a "safe" carbohydrate, such as honey, potato, sweet potato, white rice, or parsnips. Keep portion control in mind.

Carbohydrates are absolutely deadly in excess and are actually the cause behind heart disease that is misattributed to saturated fat and cholesterol. As discussed earlier in this chapter, everything from infertility and premature aging to macular degeneration can be tied to excess carbohydrate intake.

If you adopt a caveman diet in which carbohydrates are derived primarily from fruits and vegetables, it will be impossible to eat enough to hurt yourself with excess carbohydrate intake, so counting carbs will be unnecessary. If you want some root vegetables, that's fine too because they create a high level of satiety for the amount consumed. You don't *have* to eat them, but you *can*. The one thing to skip is root vegetables deep fried in industrial oils. In other words, just say "no" to french fries.

# Chapter 8
# The Deadly White Powder

Though I have addressed sugar broadly in the previous chapter by explaining how carbohydrates get converted into sugar in the body, there are specific problems with sugar *as sugar* that need to be addressed. As mentioned, the impact of the sugar within carbohydrates led to numerous health problems as we transitioned from a hunter-gatherer to an agrarian society. This occurred long before refined sugar entered the human diet on a large scale. But the introduction of refined sugar has created a whole category of problems of its own. So let's look at sugar.

## Anatomy of Sugar

Sugar refers to a class of sweet-tasting compounds consisting of single molecules (monosaccharides) or paired molecules (disaccharides). Longer chains of sugars (polysaccharides) tend to lack the characteristic sweetness of monosaccharides or disaccharides, so we call them carbohydrates or complex carbohydrates rather than sugars.

The human body doesn't directly assimilate disaccharides or polysaccharides. Instead, these are broken down into monosaccharides in the digestive tract, and it is the monosaccharides (also known as simple sugars) that are assimilated.

In nature, there are many types of monosaccharides, disaccharides, and polysaccharides. We can digest and assimilate some polysaccharides because we have enzymes that are adapted to the task. Potato and cornstarch can both be easily digested. Other polysaccharides, such as cellulose, have bonds between the sugars that are incompatible with our enzymes, so we can't digest them. Ruminant animals have gut bacteria that produce enzymes that help break them down, whereas in humans cellulose merely contributes bulk to the stool.

## Monosaccharides and Disaccharides

The most common monosaccharides in human food, either directly in the form of simple sugars or indirectly through their presence in starches or disaccharides that get broken down, are glucose (aka dextrose), fructose, and galactose. There are many other simple sugars, such as rhamnose, arabinose, raffinose, and fucose. These other simple sugars are not digestible in the small intestine and are instead broken down by fermentation bacteria in the large intestine. This is why cabbage (containing raffinose) gives some people flatulence.

Glucose, fructose, and galactose are the only simple sugars absorbed directly from the small intestine, though only glucose is directly used by the body and can be converted to energy by any cell. Fructose and galactose are converted into intermediate products identical to those made by glucose within the cells, but this is done by enzymes within the liver.

One of the hormones that controls the sense of hunger is ghrelin. As glucose levels in the blood rise in response to food, the level of ghrelin decreases, thereby signaling when it is time to stop eating. Neither fructose nor galactose affects glucose levels, hence they don't signal satiety.

In the natural world, though fructose is widely distributed, it isn't in a concentrated form. So even though eating an apple containing fructose along with other sugars might not signal satiety as quickly as it would if it contained no fructose, in practical terms it is nearly impossible to eat enough apples to be harmed.

Galactose is one of the constituents of disaccharide lactose, which is contained in milk. In people who can't digest lactose, the lactose gets fermented in the large intestine. But for infants and those who can digest lactose, it gets split into a molecule of glucose and a molecule of galactose. The galactose gets transported to the liver from the small intestine. Though lactose is used as a sweetener in some candy products and is present in sugar beets, the most likely source is milk products.

Disaccharides are formed from the combination of two simple sugars. The most common disaccharides in the human diet are sucrose (made from glucose and fructose), maltose (made from two molecules of glucose), and lactose (made from galactose and glucose). Naturally occurring foods often contain a mixture of monosaccharides and disaccharides. A pear, for example, contains glucose, fructose, and sucrose.

## Evolution and Maladaptation

In common with other modern primates, we have evolved a preference for sweet things. Long before the dawn of modern humans, it is theorized that some primates developed a sweet tooth that motivated them to pursue seasonal fruits, thereby giving them a survival advantage. As a result, those with a sweet tooth survived, and those without a sweet tooth perished.[1]

Tendencies that served us well a million or four million years ago can become maladaptive when applied within a very different environmental context. Now we live in a world awash with sugar. It is added to everything from spaghetti sauce to pickles, not to mention obvious suspects such as cookies. In this evolutionarily novel environment, our pursuit of sugar leads us to woe rather than weal.

Even though naturally occurring foods certainly contain sugars, those sugars are diluted as well as accompanied by cellulose, vegetable acids, vitamins, and minerals. For example, you'd need to eat *two pounds* of watermelon to get the same glycemic load as an ounce of table sugar! Meanwhile, you'd also be getting over 100 percent of the RDA of vitamins A and C. In our primordial environment, the pursuit of sweets was also the pursuit of a cornucopia of antioxidants, vitamins, and minerals, and the actual amount of sugar consumed was relatively small.

---

[1] R. Cohen, "Sugar Love," *National Geographic*, August 2013.

In the modern world, most items that contain sugar are processed. This means that the various ingredients have been milled, heated, filtered, purified, and otherwise rendered completely homogeneous for ease of mass production. In the process, nearly all of the natural nutritional content is destroyed or removed, and what few vitamins or minerals are to be found are added back in the form of artificial compounds. So unlike fruits or vegetables containing natural sugars, processed foods are largely nutritionally useless.

In addition, the amount of sugar added borders on the surreal. To give you an idea, a teaspoon contains four grams of sugar, or sixteen calories. A single three-ounce dessert brownie contains 45 g of carbohydrate, of which 29 g are sugar. So that tiny piece of brownie—and who can eat just one?—contains seven teaspoons of sugar.

Of course, sugar is added to a wide variety of other processed foods in order to increase their appeal. For example, a single serving of canned marinara sauce from the supermarket contains 23 g of sugar. That's right! Go read the labels at the supermarket, and you'll find brands of spaghetti sauce that contain nearly as much sugar as a decadent dessert brownie. There is so much sugar added to processed foods that the average American consumes twenty-two to twenty-eight teaspoons every day, or two *pounds* a week.[2]

And this is where maladaptive tendencies kick in. Clearly, being motivated by our genes to eat apples was very beneficial. But with everything from snack chips to cereals to salsa swimming in unnaturally high levels of sugar, it is hard for a mere apple to compete for our taste buds. This is a case where we have to employ our very large brains—also a gift of our genes—to override our desires. If we don't, the results are catastrophic.

## Dope Fiend

When most people think of drug addiction, they think of hard drugs such as heroin or cocaine along with prescription painkillers.

---

[2] J. Banks, "Hidden Sugar in Your Diet Hurting Your Health?" *Fox News*, July 10, 2013.

It's easy to associate addiction with these drugs because in the long run, the individual and social harm from their abuse is painfully evident. But part of this perception is also a matter of social norms. That is, we have decided that the harm of using cocaine is so bad it should be illegal, and as a result it is very risky to distribute. Hence, it becomes very expensive, and then a whole host of associated harms comes into play when people try to get the money to pay for the drugs.

Addictions to many other things are absolutely rampant in our society, but because these things are legal or it is easy to get prescriptions, the harmfulness isn't as apparent except in more extreme cases or when people develop chronic health problems in old age.

Alcohol and tobacco are certainly very obvious cases of legal addictive substances, but there are also a large number of prescription drugs out there (other than painkillers) that are extremely addictive. But there is one substance so deadly that, worldwide, it kills three times as many people as tobacco every year,[3] but it flies under the radar because it masquerades as a food. In terms of sheer numbers of people adversely affected, it is a larger public health threat than any illegal drug. Yes, it is sugar. Worldwide, an estimated 15,000,000 die from sugar,[4] and about 200,000 people die annually from all illegal drugs combined.[5]

Sugar is addictive. You may have heard this statement many times before, and you may sort of nod your head, but most people don't realize just how extremely addictive sugar is and how harmful the addiction can be. It kills more people than tobacco does, and the average American eats *two pounds of it a week.*

## Shooting Up

There are two mechanisms that fuel sugar addiction. The first mechanism is hormonal, and it works the same for any food

---

[3] S. Olson, "What Kills More People: Sugar or Cigarettes?" *OlsonND.com*, September 25, 2008; available at www.olsonnd.com/what-kills-more-people-sugar-or-cigarettes/.

[4] Ibid.

[5] United Nations Office on Drugs and Crime, World Drug Report 2012.

source that results in sugar uptake from the digestive tract. This particular mechanism works the same for any carbohydrate, including sugar. As your body adapts to high sugar intake, you enter a sort of "blood sugar roller coaster." Every two to four hours you feel tired, lethargic, cranky, or irritable until you eat a source of sugar, whereupon you feel fine for the next couple of hours, and the cycle repeats. Once you've climbed aboard the blood sugar roller coaster, climbing off can be very hard indeed.

The second mechanism that fuels sugar addiction is indistinguishable from the neurotransmitter and receptor changes responsible for addiction to substances such as morphine and heroin. Changes in the brain include dopamine and opioid receptor binding, enkephalin mRNA expression, and dopamine and acetylcholine release. These changes are responsible for behaviors common to drug addiction, including withdrawal, binging, and craving.[6]

A clinical review of existing research states that the mechanisms causing addiction to sugar are even more reliable at causing addiction than the mechanisms causing addiction to cocaine.

Available evidence in humans shows that sugar and sweetness can induce reward and craving that are comparable in magnitude to those induced by addictive drugs. Although this evidence is limited by the inherent difficulty of comparing different types of rewards and psychological experiences in humans, it is nevertheless supported by recent experimental research on sugar and sweet reward in laboratory rats. Overall, this research has revealed that sugar and sweet reward can not only substitute to addictive drugs, like cocaine, but can even be more rewarding and attractive. At the neurobiological level, the neural substrates of sugar and sweet reward appear to be more robust than those of cocaine (i.e., more

[6] Avena NM, Rada P, Hoebel BG. "Evidence for Sugar Addiction: Behavioral and Neurochemical Effects of Intermittent, Excessive Sugar Intake." *Neuroscience and Biobehaviorial Reviews* 2008;32(1):20-39.

resistant to functional failures), possibly reflecting past selective evolutionary pressures for seeking and taking foods high in sugar and calories.[7]

This neurotransmitter-and-receptor mechanism of addiction is related strictly to the sweet *taste* of sugar rather than the sugar itself. Because the sweet taste of artificial sweeteners can reinforce this mechanism, it is important to avoid artificial sweeteners while trying to kick sugar addiction.[8]

## The Moral Price of Sugar

Given the addictive qualities of sugar, you'd expect a major cartel or criminal enterprise to be erected around it. And you'd be right. Sugar was a primary motivating force behind the institution of slavery in the Caribbean islands following Christopher Columbus's discovery of the New World.[9, 10] One of the characteristics of serious addiction is that the addictive substance becomes so (subjectively) essential as to be a life-or-death issue for the addict, which twists the person's values in such a way that deeds that would be otherwise unacceptable seem justified.

At first blush, you are probably wondering why I'm bringing up ancient history. After all, slavery was abolished in the United States long before our great-grandparents were born. But the fact the term "slavery" is no longer applied to certain situations doesn't mean that human beings aren't being tangibly harmed. In Nicaragua, for example, thousands of sugarcane workers have died from kidney disease due to the harsh work conditions leading

---

[7] Ahmed SH, Guillem K, Vandaele Y. "Sugar addiction: Pushing the Drug-Sugar Analogy to the Limit." *Curr Opin Clin Nutr Metab Care.* 2013 Jul;16(4):434-9.

[8] Banks J. "Hidden Sugar in Your Diet Hurting Your Health?" *Fox News*, 7/10/2013

[9] Applied History Research Group, University of Calgary, 1997, *The Sugar and Slave Trades*

[10] Cohen R, "Sugar Love," *National Geographic*, August 2013

to dehydration. More men in the region die from this cause than from HIV, diabetes, and leukemia combined. The Center for Public Integrity described the phenomenon as resulting from a "legacy of neglect by industry and governments, including the United States, which have resisted pleas for aggressive action to spotlight the malady and find a remedy. Wealthier nations are more focused on spurring biofuels production in the region's sugarcane industry and keeping up the heavy flow of sugar to U.S. consumers and food manufacturers than the plight of those who harvest it."[11]

The situation in Nicaragua is far from unique. A *Fox News* article described working conditions in Brazil as "squalid" and continues as follows:

> Aside from long hours in the hot sun, cane cutters suffer a litany of bone and muscle injuries and machete cuts. Their eyes and lungs are punished by ash as they labor through fields recently burned to facilitate cutting and to kill off rats, snakes and scorpions. Some 18 cane cutters died of exhaustion in the past three years in Sao Paulo state alone, according to the Catholic Church's Migrant Workers Pastoral, which monitors working conditions. Countless others have been injured.[12]

Nearly half a million people in Brazil alone are subjected to these conditions. Thousands have died in Nicaragua. I'm just scratching the surface because this is a book on diet instead of world affairs, but this should be enough data to see that the pure white crystals in the sugar jar are tarnished with the blood of human suffering. It comes at a moral cost.

I should note in fairness that organic, Fair Trade-certified sugar guarantees that workers have access to water, shade, rest breaks, education, and health care. It's more expensive, but health

---

[11] R. Greene, "Thousands of Sugar Cane Workers Die as Wealthy Nations Stall on Solutions," *The Center for Public Integrity*, December 12, 2011.

[12] "Harsh Working Conditions in Brazil Show Dark Side of Ethanol Production," *Fox News/Associated Press*, October 2, 2007

concerns indicate you shouldn't be using sugar much (or even at all) anyway. So you should be avoiding sugar in the first place, but if you decide to buy it anyway—say, to make a sculpture or something—get the organic stuff.

## Dental Problems, Revisited

The previous chapter on carbohydrates documented clear harm from their overconsumption, including metabolic disorder, cardiovascular disease, increased risk of cancer, and even depression and anxiety. Carbohydrates in general need to be strictly regulated to avoid harm. But the reason carbohydrates have these adverse affects is that they turn into sugar in the intestines. Therefore, all of the harms that result from carbohydrates are also attributable to sugars. But in addition to addiction, concentrated sugars bring unique harms.

As we explored in the chapter on grains, I mentioned that it was the addition of grain to the modern human diet that introduced humans to tooth decay. The proportion of people in society afflicted with tooth decay went from less than 1 percent to more than 20 percent. But sugar kicks this into overdrive.

The bacteria responsible for tooth decay cannot digest the complex carbohydrates in grains directly. Instead, they live on the small amount of sugar created by the interaction between carbohydrates and the ptyalin in saliva. But when you dump seven teaspoons of pure sugar into your mouth with grandma's delicious brownies, you might as well sign your paycheck over to the dentist. Even though the introduction of grain into the human diet brought us 20 percent of people having cavities, things get even worse. According to the National Institutes of Health, with our current system buried in sugar, 92 percent of adults have tooth decay, and the average adult has three or four rotted or missing teeth.[13]

---

[13] National Health and Nutrition Examination Survey, 1999–2004.

## Hormones, Gallstones, and Gout—Oh, My!

Sugar—specifically glucose, fructose, and sucrose—when used in excess of levels found in natural foods, has also been demonstrated to turn off certain genes in the liver regulating sex hormones.[14] If you're a man and you have sore nipples, it's the estradiol (a powerful form of estrogen) you are making from eating sugar.[15] Would you like some more cake? Sugar consumption also causes gallstones,[16] kidney stones,[17, 18] and gout.[19] The harms of sugar are so varied and extensive that several books have been written about that topic alone, but the most dangerous aspect of sugar is its role in cancer.

## Sugar, Immunity, and Cancer

Sugar—fructose particularly, which is contained in table sugar and most concentrated sugars—also weakens your immune system when consumed in excess. Specifically, the ability of immune cells to engulf and destroy invaders (such as bacteria) is substantially inhibited for up to five hours after consuming sugar.[20] In addition, high fructose consumption induces inflammation generally

---

[14] G. Hammond *et al.*, "Monosaccharide-Induced Lipogenesis Regulates the Human Hepatic Sex Hormone Binding Globulin Gene," *Journal of Clinical Investigation* 117 (2007): 3979–87.

[15] J. Yudkin and O. Eisa, "Dietary Sucrose and Oestradiol Concentration in Young Men." *Annals of Nutrition and Metabolism* 32, no. 2 (1988): 53–55.

[16] K. W. Heaton, "The Epidemiology of Gallstones and Suggested Aetiology," *Clinical Gastroenterology* 2, no. 1 (1973): 67–83.

[17] N. J. Blacklock, "Sucrose and Idiopathic Renal Stone," *Nutrition and Health* 5, nos. 1–2 (1987): 9–12.

[18] G. Curhan *et al.*, "Beverage Use and Risk for Kidney Stones in Women," *Annals of Internal Medicine* 28 (1998): 534–40.

[19] X. Gao *et al.*, "Intake of Added Sugar and Sugar-Sweetened Drink and Serum Uric Acid Concentration in US Men and Women," *Hypertension* 50, no. 2 (2007): 306–12.

[20] A. Sanches *et al.*, "Role of Sugars in Human Neutrophilic Phagocytosis," *American Journal of Clinical Nutrition* 26 no. 11 (1973): 1180–84.

throughout the body,[21] leading to a wide variety of maladies, including predisposing a wide variety of cancers.[22] Recent research has demonstrated *how* sugar predisposes cancer. In general, if a cell is damaged or mutates, it commits suicide (a process called apoptosis) rather than pose a risk to the body as a whole. Likewise, normal cells can only divide a finite number of times. Chromosomes have telomere tails that are required for replication. These get shorter each time they replicate, until they aren't long enough to divide.

In cancer cells, the telomeres don't get shorter with each division, and though apoptosis can be forced through extraordinary damage (by using radiation or chemotherapy drugs for example), the threshold is much higher than in a normal cell. Thus, cancer cells are effectively immortal. It is this immortality that makes cancer cells cancerous. Without the element of immortality, the damage that a mutated cell can do is extremely limited, and the cell will usually commit suicide anyway. At worst, it results in a benign tumor that can be surgically removed, and no further problems ensue.

The key role played by sugar in cancer, and why it predisposes so many seemingly unrelated types of cancer, is that it turns on the "immortality switch." Though it has been known for some time that diabetes, obesity, and cancer all tend to run together and that high sugar consumption is associated with increased cancer risk, the mechanism for this was unknown. It was accidentally discovered by a group of scientists researching the interaction between intestinal cells and insulin.

High sugar levels lead to the accumulation of a protein called beta-catenin in the nucleus of cells, and it is this accumulation that turns on the immortality switch, making cancer possible. Though the language is a bit technical, the scientists summarized the matter beautifully.

---

[21] Y. Rayssiguier *et al.*, "High Fructose Consumption Combined with Low Dietary Magnesium Intake May Increase the Incidence of the Metabolic Syndrome by Inducing Inflammation," *Magnesium Research* 19, no. 4 (2006): 237–43.

[22] S. Rakoff-Nahoum, "Why Cancer and Inflammation?" *Yale Journal of Biology and Medicine* 79, nos. 3–4 (2006): 123–30.

Nuclear accumulation of β-catenin, a widely recognized marker of poor cancer prognosis, drives cancer cell proliferation and senescence bypass and regulates incretins, critical regulators of fat and glucose metabolism. . . . Here, we show that high glucose is essential for nuclear localization of β-catenin in response to Wnt signaling. . . . Consequently β-catenin accumulates in the nucleus and activates target promoters under combined glucose and Wnt stimulation, but not with either stimulus alone. Our results reveal a mechanism by which high glucose enhances signaling through the cancer-associated Wnt/β-catenin pathway.[23]

Not only does sugar consumption predispose cancers but also once the cancer is under way, sugar feeds the cancer it created.[24, 25] Elevated sugar consumption also plays a critical role in encouraging cancers to spread.[26] In fact, though it is not yet widely used in cancer treatment, a ketogenic diet high in fat, moderate in protein, and very low in carbohydrate shows considerable promise in treating cancer.[27, 28] This is not at all surprising given that cancer cells have a compromised metabolism that can use glucose only for energy, whereas ordinary (noncancerous) cells can use ketone

---

[23] C. Garcia-Jimenez *et al.*, "Glucose-Induced β-Catenin Acetylation Enhances Wnt Signaling in Cancer," *Molecular Cell* 49, no. 3 (2012): 474–86.

[24] T. Volk *et al.*, "pH in Human Tumor Xenografts: Effect of Intravenous Administration of Glucose," *British Journal of Cancer* 68, no. 3 (1993): 492–500.

[25] F. Rossi-Fanelli *et al.*, "Abnormal Substrate Metabolism and Nutritional Strategies in Cancer Management," *Journal of Parenteral and Enteral Nutrition* 15, no. 6 (1991): 680–83.

[26] R. Gillies, I. Robey, and R. Gatenby, "Causes and Consequences of Increased Glucose Metabolism in Cancers," *Journal of Nuclear Medicine* 49 suppl 2 (2008): 24S–42S.

[27] B. A. Simone *et al.*, "Selectively Starving Cancer Cells Through Dietary Manipulation: Methods and Clinical Implications," *Future Oncology* 9, no. 7 (2013): 959–76.

[28] B. G. Allen *et al.*, "Ketogenic Diets Enhance Oxidative Stress and Radio-Chemo-Therapy Responses in Lung Cancer Xenografts," *Clinical Cancer Research* 19, no. 14 (2013): 3905–13.

bodies as an alternative fuel. Dr. Tomas Seyfried has advanced the idea of cancer, in general, being a metabolic disorder caused by bad diet (too much aggregate sugar) and that cancer can be prevented and managed through diet. Key aspects of management include caloric restriction and a ketogenic diet.[29]

The bottom line is that a host of nasty cancers all share a common link with sugar consumption as a predisposing factor. But if you want to prevent cancer, avoiding excessive carbohydrates generally and concentrated sugars in particular is a winning strategy.

## Identifying Sugar Addiction

When transitioning to a caveman diet, people usually have no trouble giving up legumes, only a little trouble giving up grains, and no real difficulty giving up dairy or industrial oils. But it is very common for people to have trouble giving up sugar. Because concentrated sugars such as honey are allowed in moderation, a very common problem is for people to substitute honey and other concentrated sugars for the calories they were previously deriving from grains.

No! No! No! Moderation does *not* mean you get to eat concentrated sugars daily, pig out on your favorite ice cream, and so forth. It means that of the twenty-one meals you eat weekly, only *three* of them can include a concentrated sweetener—preferably unpasteurized honey. That's it. No more.

This moderation tends to be a problem because of sugar addiction. Sugar addiction, like any other addiction, is a complex phenomenon. In the case of sugar, it entails three aspects. In each individual who is addicted to sugar, the three aspects will be present in varying degrees, though one aspect is usually dominant over the others.

---

[29] T. Seyfried, *Cancer as a Metabolic Disease: On the Origin, Management and Prevention of Cancer* (Hoboken: John Wiley, 2012).

Sugar addiction has a psychological aspect. People associate sugar as a reward and will treat themselves to something sugary in response to various stresses. Thus, strong psychological associations are made akin to conditioned responses. People who reward themselves with candy or cookies after completing a difficult task or who use sweet treats as a refuge from emotional turmoil are stereotypical of this form of sugar addiction.

The hormonal aspect of sugar addiction encompasses insulin resistance, leptin resistance, and the blood sugar roller coaster. The hormonal aspect of sugar addiction can be satisfied by any easily broken down carbohydrate, so you don't need cookies or candy to satisfy it—chips, pretzels, popcorn, and similar foods will meet the need just fine. You know you are dealing with the roller coaster if you find yourself needing something sweet or crunchy (and carrots won't do!) or a "snack" every two to four hours in order to avoid feeling lethargic, irritable, unable to concentrate, or otherwise out of sorts.

The blood sugar roller coaster is often referred to as hypoglycemia, though what most people are experiencing doesn't meet the medical definition for that diagnosis. The medical definition for that diagnosis requires that blood sugar levels be below normal, and clinical acute hypoglycemia of that sort is a life-threatening situation. The "hypoglycemia" that most people are referring to doesn't really result in clinically measurable lower-than-normal levels of blood sugar. It is, however, a prelude to developing insulin resistance and is a very real phenomenon. It is hard to measure in a clinical setting, so doctors don't really know exactly what is going on, but the behavior and cravings are obvious, and anyone who has ever experienced the phenomenon can relate to what I'm describing.

Leptin resistance is another hormonal aspect of sugar addiction. The systems for signaling satiety or when to stop eating are complex and interrelated, but leptin is a master hormone signaling how many calories your body needs. Leptin is created by fat cells and picked up by the hypothalamus in the brain. Excessive fat tissue makes too much leptin, forcing the receptors for leptin to down-regulate, so they are less sensitive. Then, it becomes a vicious cycle: You always feel hungry, and you can literally eat to the point of physical discomfort before considering yourself to be full. It is very difficult for people with leptin resistance to diet, because they feel hungry unless sated to a very high degree. How does the cycle get started in the first place? If lectins from grains enter the blood stream, they can block the leptin receptors.[30] Unable to realize you are full, your appetite becomes disregulated, you add fat cells, and then the vicious cycle begins.

Doctors will typically use a combination of blood tests and a bit of observation to diagnose leptin resistance. The symptoms are varied and depressing. In women, it can resemble polycystic ovarian syndrome: infertility, abnormal menstrual cycles, androgen production, and facial hair growth. It also causes fatigue and insomnia. These symptoms can make it difficult to engage in exercise or change diet.

Insulin resistance is another component of the hormonal aspect of sugar addiction. Doctors will diagnose it officially using a glucose tolerance test, but you are likely to be insulin resistant if your waist circumference is greater than forty inches for a man or thirty-five inches for a woman. Researchers are still delving into the mechanisms of insulin resistance, but there is little doubt as to the cause: chronic consumption of excess sugars or carbohydrates that readily turn into sugars in the digestive tract. Over time, insulin receptors in the cells require higher and higher levels of insulin in order to respond, meanwhile leaving levels of blood sugar elevated.

The third aspect of sugar addiction is brain physiology. Sugar addiction (actually, sweetness addiction) makes changes in the neurotransmitters and receptors in the brain similar to those made by heroin or morphine. A clear indication of these changes in the brain can be seen in cravings for "something sweet." While the affected person may have a preference for a particular sweet,

---

[30] Y. Kamikubo *et al.*, "Contribution of Leptin Receptor N-Linked Glycans to Leptin Binding," *Biochemical Journal* 410, no. 3 (2008): 595–604.

if the sweet of choice is unavailable, anything sweet will do. Another clear indication is gorging on sweets after a short period of deprivation.

Not everyone addicted to sugar has all of these aspects of the addiction, but which aspects are predominant for a given individual make a difference in strategies for kicking the habit.

## Kicking the Psychological Addiction

In general, this aspect of sugar addiction is the easiest to overcome. Though most people have a general awareness that "sugar is bad," they aren't really aware of how incredibly bad it is. Once the true physical dangers of sugar are understood, it becomes increasingly hard to see sweets as a reward. ("Wow, Brett, you did a great job on that project! Reward yourself with some tooth decay, diabetes, heart disease, and cancer!") When concentrated sugars are seen as being the *true threats to health that they really are*, they lose their luster as a reward.

It's also hard to see sugar as a reward when you know that people are laboring in such poor working conditions that they are literally dying by the thousands in order to put cheap sugar in your treats. A piece of candy loses its allure when you realize that someone may have died from exhaustion to provide the main ingredient: sugar. Though these moral concerns can be addressed by using local honey, maple syrup, or sugar made using humane employment, the health concerns of excess usage remain.

In aggregate, however, the health and moral concerns, once truly acknowledged and understood, are sufficient to address the psychological aspects of the addiction for most people. If that is insufficient in a particular case, the psychological aspects of sugar addiction are addressable through hypnosis.[31]

---

[31] New York Hypnosis Institute, "Eliminate Sugar Cravings Hypnosis"; available at www.tryhypnosisnow.com/eliminate-sugar-cravings-hypnosis-nyc/.

## Kicking the Hormonal Addiction

For people who are of normal weight or no more than fifty pounds overweight, the hormonal aspects of sugar addiction can usually be addressed without professional assistance. If, however, blood tests show you to be diabetic or prediabetic, or you are obese rather than overweight, you may benefit from certain drugs a physician will prescribe to help with leptin resistance and insulin resistance. The drugs are not miracles—they are no substitute for the rest of what is needed—but they will help make pursuing the correct course of action easier.

All hormonal aspects of addiction to sugar can be addressed through diet and exercise. A caveman diet as specified in this book will do just fine. The only necessary modification for dealing with the blood sugar roller coaster is to divide your meals into several smaller meals or to make sure you have good snacks available every couple of hours.

The big thing you'll need to watch is your total daily glycemic load. As I described in the previous chapter, when following a caveman diet, you don't usually need to keep track. But when dealing with sugar addiction, adhering to daily glycemic load limits is critical, so you should get a glycemic load chart (or find one on the Internet—there are several) and write down the glycemic load of everything you eat. You want your total glycemic load for the day to stay under the glycemic load for five slices of white bread. The reason I don't provide a number is because glycemic load charts vary. So, if you look up the glycemic load for a slice of white bread in your reference chart and multiply it by five, it will work perfectly with whatever chart you are using.

Make sure you have some protein every time you eat, even if it is just a snack. You can make some hard-boiled eggs and bring three of them with you to work. Have one with each snack. Bring a package of salmon. Pack a rib eye. Whatever it takes, make sure you have protein. Also, don't skimp on the fat. When it comes to dealing with the hormonal aspects of sugar addiction, natural fats are your friend. At the end of each time you eat, have a piece of fruit (*real* fruit, no dehydrated fruits allowed until you've broken the addiction). Fish is important because the omega-3 fats in fish help to reestablish insulin sensitivity.

You need to get your sleep. If you find your sleep less than restful, get checked for sleep apnea (especially if you are substantially overweight). If you need a special machine or a prosthesis to make sure your airway stays unobstructed through the night, use it, and you won't be sorry. Leptin interacts with cortisol levels from excessive stress and insufficient sleep, and getting your sleep will make correcting leptin resistance problems much easier.

Even though you may wish to lose weight, and most people lose weight anyway when they undertake a caveman diet, don't try to restrict your calories when trying to break sugar addiction. That's because serious caloric restriction can keep the fat cells in your body from making leptin. If you know you are leptin resistant, limit your fruit intake to three fruits daily until your leptin resistance is fixed, because fructose causes your liver to generate trigylcerides that block leptin.

Meanwhile, undertake an exercise program like the one I describe later in this book. The program I describe will also improve your blood sugar control. It can be done in your own home in little time and will also increase your metabolism. If you work better in a group setting, just find a CrossFit gym near you. CrossFit is very similar to the interval-based techniques I have described, but it is group-based and has very supportive members and qualified staff to help you. CrossFit adapts to your level of fitness, whatever it is when you start, and then grows with you. If all you know of Crossfit is what you see on TV, it may appear to be suitable only for people with superhero physiques. But Crossfit has an "on-ramp" program and specific protocols for adapting exercises for people who are sedentary, obese, etc.

I wish I could tell you that you only have to follow this program for a week, but the cold reality is that you'll have to do it for four to six weeks or until your waist size is under forty inches (for men) or thirty-five inches (for women). Once you are at that point, you can switch to three meals a day (plus snacks) rather than multiple small meals, and you can eat as much fruit as you'd like—though

I still caution against any more than a quarter of a cup of dehydrated fruits a day.

## Kicking the Physiological Brain Addiction

For the neurotransmitter aspects of sugar addiction, you will need to avoid all concentrated sweeteners, including artificial sweeteners (even in gum), until your neurotransmitters and receptors have rebalanced. There aren't any studies on how long this takes in the case of sugar addiction, but since the mechanisms are similar to those present in opioid addiction, the timeline is likely similar.

In cases of opioid addiction, within a month neurotransmitters and receptors are 45 to 50 percent back to normal. How long it takes to recover completely beyond that varies substantially between individuals, with the time ranging from six months to a year. The first month is the hardest part.

Fruits are not concentrated sweeteners, but they are definitely sweet. Using them in place of concentrated sweeteners (such as by using a piece of fruit for dessert rather than a candy bar) will gradually wean you off of concentrated sugars.

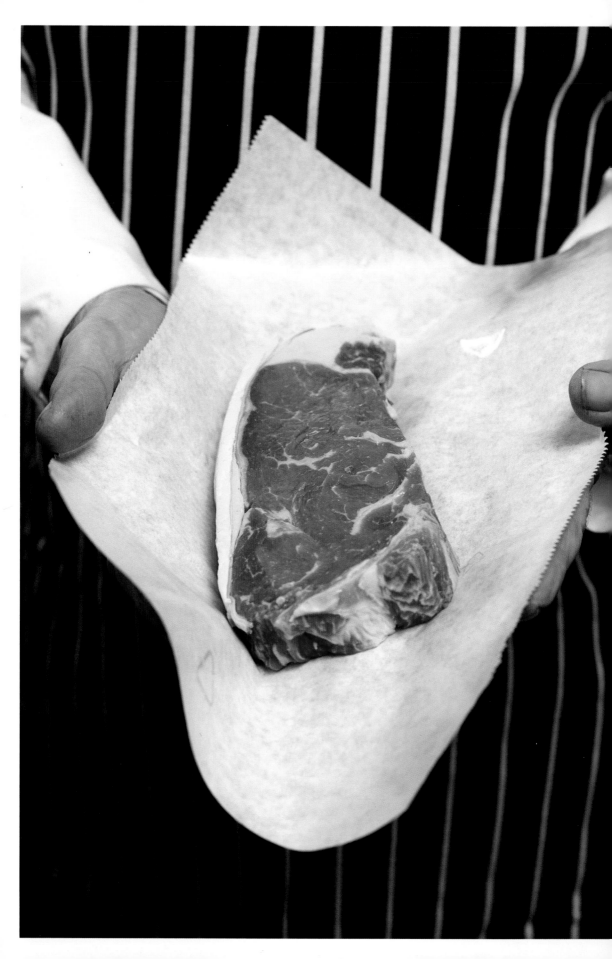

# Chapter 9
# Meat's Back on the Menu

Throughout this book I have discussed the detrimental aspects of vegetable sources of protein, such as legumes and grains, as well as the costs and benefits of dairy. It should be clear at this point that the healthiest sources of protein in the diet are meat (from land and sea) and eggs—and this is where our caveman ancestors got their protein as well. In fact, it is the adoption of sea and land animals as dietary staples that allowed our ancestors to evolve the large brains that define us as human.[1]

Protein is a series of amino acids linked together, and so amino acids are the building blocks of our genetic code and life itself. An amino acid has a "-COOH" group on one end, just like a fatty acid. But in addition, it has an "-NH$_2$" group on that end as well. The rest of it is made up of a wide variety of possible structures. About 500 amino acids are known. Of all the amino acids, twenty-three are able to form into chains to create proteins. It is the length of the chains and the sequence of amino acids in the chains that make each protein unique. The number of possible combinations is effectively infinite.

The human body is able to synthesize some amino acids, but others are called "essential" because the body can't manufacture them. Essential amino acids have to be derived from diet in the form of ingested proteins.

All living things contain protein because the very DNA within the nucleus of their cells is composed of protein. Though the mix of amino acids differs, in theory, if you eat enough of practically anything, you can get enough of the essential amino acids. Also,

---

[1] C. L. Broadhurst *et al.*, "Brain-Specific Lipids from Marine, Lacustrine, or Terrestrial Food Resources: Potential Impact on Early African Homo Sapien," *Comparative Biochemistry and Physiology Part B: Biochemistry and Molecular Biology* 131 (2002):653–73.

some foods may be relatively deficient in some amino acids in which another food has abundance—so combining those foods to get the right mix will reduce the total amount of food that needs to be consumed to get the required amino acids. In addition, these foods don't have to be combined within a single meal—we have a twenty-four-hour window during which the combination can be achieved.

The foregoing information will be of particular value to vegans. Unfortunately, the only foods a vegan can eat that have sufficient protein concentrations to even be considered as replacements for meat are foods that should be avoided for other reasons, such as grains and legumes. In theory, it is possible to render these foods safe through a process of sprouting and fermentation, but this isn't practical for people living modern lifestyles governed by a clock. It is also possible for a person to get enough essential amino acids from potatoes if they were the only item in the diet. But the downsides of such a high-carbohydrate diet were discussed in the previous chapter: heart disease, increased cancer risk, metabolic syndrome, and infertility among many others.

Raw veganism in particular is a very good short-term *detoxifying* diet to help people recover from eating industrial garbage. As I mentioned previously, practically any diet, even veganism, will provide at least temporary benefits compared to the standard American diet consisting of buckets of processed "food." French fries made in industrial oils shipped by tanker truck, fluorescent orange powdered "cheese" reconstituted with canola, FD&C green, brominated vegetable oil, meats preserved with potassium nitrite, and cheese doodles aren't even *food* by any sensible definition.

It's obvious that any diet that induces someone to throw that trash in the garbage where it belongs and actually *eat some vegetables for a change* will bring enormous benefits. But vegan-type diets are strictly for the short term. They can help *detoxify* when used wisely for a very short time period (of a month or less), but they cannot *nourish.*

Recently, a French mother whose breast milk was deficient in essential vitamins due to her vegan diet was sentenced to five years in prison because her baby died as a result.[2] There was another case in Atlanta of committed vegans killing their baby by feeding it soy and fruit juice. Then there was the twelve-year-old boy in Scotland whose vegan diet had him bound to a wheelchair and hopelessly deformed for life. You can use any search engine and find dozens of cases of children being harmed in numerous ways from vegan diets. Though it may be theoretically possible to maintain a healthy vegan diet, the reality of trying to do this in a world governed by a time clock and financial constraints is far different. Even the vegan girlfriend of Morgan Spurlock (famous for his documentary *Super Size Me*) and celebrity vegan Ellen Degeneres eventually had to drop veganism.

As the chapters of this book have laid out in detail and with copious citations of peer-reviewed studies, any diet that has grains and legumes as usually prepared or anything else high in carbohydrates as its basis is ultimately incompatible with a long and healthy life. The same goes for diets high in vegetable oils. The human body was designed to eat meat, it is meat that literally made us human, and it is upon meat that your body will thrive.

## Omega-6 and Omega-3 Levels in Meat

The importance of maintaining a ratio of omega-6 to omega-3 polyunsaturated fats in the diet was covered in the chapter on fats. This becomes relevant with regard to meat because modern confinement meat production operations generate meat that is higher in omega-6 than the wild meats available during most of our evolution.

One way to solve this problem is to raise meat and eggs yourself or become a very proficient hunter. For my family growing up, both served as the predominant sources of meat, and I still hunt

---

[2] "Baby Breastfed By Vegan Mother Dies," *The Healthy Home Economist*, March 30, 2011; available at www.thehealthyhomeeconomist.com/baby-breastfed-by-vegan-mother-dies/.

and raise some of my own meat and eggs. But this isn't practical for someone living in a 400 sq. ft. studio apartment in Brooklyn.

Another option is to purchase grass-fed, free-range, and organic eggs and meat. These types of meat have superior levels of omega-3 fats, and they don't contribute added hormones and antibiotics to the food supply. Unfortunately, grass-fed, organic, and free-range meat and eggs tend to be expensive—roughly three times the cost of their industrial equivalents. If you can afford these—excellent; please do so. But what if you can't?

If you can't, don't worry. Free-range eggs are affordable. You can buy wild-caught fish that was frozen at sea (and also canned varieties), and canned sardines in water are also affordable. All three of these items are very high in omega-3, and if you eat fish just three times a week, it is sufficient to balance out the omega-6 from industrial meat. Let's look at an eight-ounce serving of industrially produced T-bone steak.

An eight-ounce portion of T-bone steak has 16 g of saturated fat, 21 g of monounsaturated fat, and 1.6 g of polyunsaturated fat. The saturated fat has no adverse effects, the monounsaturated fat has the same benefits as the monounsaturated fat in olive oil, and the amount of polyunsaturated fat is so small that even if it were all omega-6, it would be balanced out by only a quarter of a can of sardines.

Along with this you'd get 53 g of complete protein, 117 percent of the RDA of vitamin B12, 106 percent of the RDA for selenium, 96 percent of the RDA of zinc, 69 percent of the RDA of niacin, 59 percent of the RDA of vitamin B6, and so forth. And that is industrial feedlot beef. Grass-fed beef is even more nutritious. But feedlot beef, included in the diet daily, has a favorable effect on blood lipids and reduces markers of inflammation when trimmed of visible fat.[3]

How about a couple of pork chops? Two pork chops (using data from industrial feedlot pork—free-range pork is more healthy) deliver

---

[3] M. A. Roussell E *et al.*, "Beef in an Optimal Lean Diet Study: Effects on Lipids, Lipoproteins, and Apolipoproteins," *American Journal of Clinical Nutrition* 95, no. 1 (2012): 9–16.

7 g of saturated fat, 8 g of monounsaturated fat, and 2.4 g of poly-unsaturated fat. (Even if all of it is omega-6, it would take only half of a can of sardines to balance it out. I use sardines as an example, but other fish would work fine.) It also gives you 31 g of complete protein, 104 percent of the RDA for thiamine, 40 percent of the RDA of phosphorus, 38 percent of the RDA of riboflavin, and more.

I deliberately picked fatty cuts of meat to make a point: that though the worse omega-6 ratio of modern meats is regrettable, it makes up such a small portion of the total fat in meat that it can be very easily balanced with some salmon, tuna, sardines, anchovies, or other seafood that it isn't a problem.

Furthermore, what I just described is a worst-case scenario. Instead of eating pork chops, you could choose tenderloin, and instead of a T-bone steak, you could choose top round—both of which are much lower in total fat. The fat in meat is good for you, but choosing lean cuts will still give you plenty of fat without doubling down on excessive caloric intake. In terms of weight, it isn't just what you eat that matters but also the amount that you eat.

## Hormones in Feedlot Beef and Sheep

I would prefer meat that hasn't been subjected to outside hormonal interference, simply because there are limits to human knowledge and there could certainly be a "gotcha" that I've missed. But my research indicates that residual hormone levels are not a problem in meats so long as the hormonal implants are used as specified by law. Human knowledge will always be imperfect, and this factor is compounded by both the involvement of parties with a vested interest as well as the legendary corruption of regulatory agencies.[4] Even so, my honest assessment of current knowledge is that the hormone implants in meat (they are used only in cattle and sheep, not in pigs, dairy cattle, or chickens) aren't a problem so long as they are used in accordance with established protocols.

---

[4] For a rundown on regulatory corruption in general, please see www.open-secrets.org.

Animal tissues naturally contain hormones, such as progesterone, estradiol, and testosterone. How much of these hormones they contain varies with the age and sex of the animal, whether it is pregnant/nursing, or if it has been spayed or neutered. This applies both to ourselves and to the animals we eat. Livestock implants are usually of testosterone, estrogen, and progesterone (which are naturally occurring), or of the artificial hormones zeranol and trenbolone. Some implants contain a mixture. These implants raise the level of hormones in the livestock to h igher levels than they would otherwise have naturally, in order to make them gain weight faster but also be leaner. The implant is placed just behind an ear, and that area is trimmed and discarded during processing.

For any substance, there is a threshold of dosage below which it has no discernible effect. For example, apple seeds contain a cyanogenic glycoside that turns into deadly cyanide gas in the stomach. The reason why nobody has ever dropped dead from eating an incidental apple seed is that our body has an innate capacity to detoxify cyanide, and it isn't until the dosage of cyanide exceeds our body's capacity for detoxification that adverse symptoms are observed. Hormones are no different in that there is a dosage below which there are no discernible effects, because the body clears them as fast as they come in.

For something such as cyanide that isn't normally present in the body, it is pretty easy to tell if any cyanide that is present is the result of eating a particular item, because all the cyanide in the body doesn't belong there. With hormones the matter is more difficult because animal foods all contain hormones naturally, and humans also contain hormones naturally. Usually, the amount of hormones in a person is so great, and assimilation from the digestive tract so poor, that it is like ascertaining which portion of a bowling ball is contributed by a pea. Matters are made even more complex by the fact that many foods, such as dairy and even potatoes, contain extremely high hormone levels naturally. Separating the effects of a steak and a potato with butter eaten at the same meal is difficult without completely controlling someone's diet.

The units used for measuring hormone levels in meat are so small (on the order of nanograms or picograms per kilogram of meat) that it is hard for people to assign meaning to the numbers. And, really, because hormones are so powerful in their effects, describing these units of measurement could be deceptive. So, instead, I am going to give a few hard numbers but primarily describe ratios as they give a basis for comparison.

The FDA has established thresholds for hormones in humans below which they are believed to have no effect. It is not possible to have 100 percent certainty in this knowledge because in order to get perfect data, we'd have to use humans of various population groups as test subjects, remove their sex organs so they didn't produce the hormones themselves, and then test with progressive doses over a long period of time until effects were observed. So far, the politicians who should have volunteered as test subjects have held out, so the data we have is based upon both indirect measurements in humans (usually testing of hormone replacement therapies in older men and women) and tests on animals (including primates) who have been spayed or neutered. Like I said, the resulting knowledge is not perfect, but the studies seem quite reasonable.

The NHEL (no hormonal effect level) for estradiol is 5 µg per kilogram of bodyweight. The NHEL for progesterone is 3.3 mg per kilogram of bodyweight. The NHEL for testosterone is 1.7 mg per kilogram of bodyweight. So if you weigh 150 lbs, you would see no effect from 341 µg of estradiol, 225 mg of progesterone, and 116 mg of testosterone.[5] Based on this, the acceptable daily intake (ADI) of these was set at .05, 30, and 2 µg per kilogram of bodyweight, respectively. For a 150 lbs person, this works out to 3.4 µg of estradiol, 2 mg of progesterone, and 136 µg of testosterone daily. As a point of reference, these numbers were set with a very large margin of safety because the limit for estradiol is 1 percent of the NHEL, the limit for progesterone is less than 1 percent of the NHEL, and the limit for testosterone is less than one-tenth of 1 percent of the NHEL.

---

[5] Joint FAO/WHO Expert Committee on Food Additives, "Summary and Conclusions of the Fifty-second Meeting," Rome, February 2–11, 1999.

The natural levels of various hormones are different for calves, bulls, steers, and heifers. Rather than break this down exhaustively for each hormone for each type of cattle and whether or not the cattle were implanted, I am instead going to provide the average concentration of each hormone in meat both with and without hormone implant.

|  | Without Implant | With Implant |
|---|---|---|
| Estradiol: | 8.6 pg/g | 11 pg/g |
| Progesterone: | 0.59 mg/kg | 0.67 mg/kg |
| Testosterone: | 0.10 mg/kg | 0.11 mg/kg |

These numbers may be putting you to sleep, so let me quickly summarize this by translating all these units into something sensible. What does this mean if you sit down and eat a pound of steak that has been treated with an implant versus a pound of steak that has not been treated with an implant? The difference is so small as to be statistically insignificant and certainly is well below the NHEL by a factor of hundreds. To put these numbers in perspective, skim milk has 2.2 mg of estradiol per liter (which is ironically well beyond the ADI), butter has 4.2 mg of progesterone per tablespoon, and cheese can have as much as 0.04 mg of testosterone per ounce—ten times as much as the difference between eating a pound of implanted versus nonimplanted beef.[6, 7]

In other words, this is a nonissue. If you are concerned about exogenous hormones in your diet, legumes contain far more than implanted cattle. For example, you will get 113,500,000 ng of estrogens from a pound of tofu versus 7 ng of estrogens from a pound of implanted beef.[8]

---

[6] The numbers in this section were taken from research performed by Ellin Doyle at the Food Research Institute at the University of Wisconsin. My numbers do not directly quote the numbers in Dr. Doyle's report but instead represent the use of averaging, extensive unit conversions, and extrapolation. Therefore, though the research credit goes to Dr. Doyle, I am personally responsible for the numbers in this section.

[7] E. Doyle, "Human Safety of Hormone Implants Used to Promote Growth in Cattle," Food Research Institute, University of Wisconsin, 2000.

[8] F. Stoler, "Hormones in Cows and What It Means for Your Health," *Fox News*, March 30, 2012.

If you can afford it and if you have a choice, by all means go for grass-fed, free-range, organic meat. It *is* healthier. But don't let fear of hormones in meat drive you to far more dangerous alternatives.

## Antibiotics in Livestock Operations

Millions of pounds of antibiotics are used in livestock operations annually, mostly as a preventative measure because livestock are confined in conditions that are ideal for the development and spread of disease. It is a perfect case of going against nature and then using something unnatural to fix the problems that wouldn't exist in the first place if livestock were being raised in a more natural way. From a long-range and environmental perspective, this can't be good.

If you want to know why this is happening, it is because of the nature of commodity markets. In a commodity market, there is no recognition of added value for a product raised humanely or in better conditions. Pork bellies are pork bellies. The exception is organic produce, which trades as a separate commodity. But even there, the pressure is always to cut costs because it is always possible for the market price of an item to be less than the cost of raising it. Until the fundamental nature of markets can be changed, there will always be issues like this. As I write this, wages for most people have remained stagnant for at least a decade relative to inflation, so it isn't as though there are people standing in line volunteering to pay double or triple the price of food commodities for better products. There is a reason why the section for grass-fed beef at the supermarket where I shop is literally one foot wide. Though the market for superior products *is* growing, it is still very small compared with the overall market.

But back to antibiotics in livestock, the real question from a dietary perspective is whether there are residues sufficient to make them unwise to eat. Just as with hormones, extensive testing has been done to ascertain the no observable effect level (NOEL) for antibiotics, and the acceptable tissue levels in processed livestock are mandated to be about a thousandth of this level. Because antibiotics are naturally metabolized and eliminated, there is a mandatory withdrawal period for antibiotics prior to processing, and during that time the level of antibiotics in tissues falls well below the mandated level due to ordinary metabolic processes. Certain antibiotics are metabolized too slowly for this, and these antibiotics are illegal to use.

A four-year review of residue level compliance in poultry found 100 percent compliance during two of the four years, 99.8 percent compliance during one year, and 99.8 percent compliance with chickens and 99.6 percent compliance with turkeys in the remaining year. Even those small areas of noncompliance were within the margin of a 100-fold safety factor.[9]

When it comes to beef and pork, though, the picture isn't as rosy. Every week the USDA publishes a list of repeat offenders whose residues exceed maximums more than once in a one-year period. The list published on July 4, 2013, is seventeen pages long and includes some cases in which residues were ten times the level allowed.[10] This demonstrates that there is a pervasive culture within the industry of producers who skirt the laws and do not care if their products are safe so long as they can sell them.

To make matters worse, though some veterinary drugs (such as penicillin) are destroyed by standard cooking methods, others (such as nitroimidazole drugs) are very stable when exposed to heat, so they are not destroyed even by thorough cooking.[11] Another study on residues of oxytetracycline, streptomycin, and other common veterinary antibiotics found that the effect of cooking and cold storage ranged from minimal to nil.[12]

---

[9] D. J. Donoghue, "Antibiotic Residues in Poultry Tissues and Eggs: Human Health Concerns?" *Poultry Science* 82, no. 4 (2003): 618–21.

[10] FSIS Residue Violation Information System, "Weekly Residue Repeat Violator Report," July 4, 2013.

[11] M. Rose, J. Bygrave, and M. Sharman, "Effect of Cooking on Veterinary Drug Residues," Parts 8 and 9, *Analyst* 122 (1997): 1095–99; 124 (1999): 289–94.

[12] J. J. O'Brien, N. Campbell, and T. Conaghan, "Effect of Cooking and Cold Storage on Biologically Active Antibiotic Residues in Meat," *Journal of Hygiene* (London) 87, no. 3 (1981):511–23.

Because you can't count on cooking to destroy antibiotic residues and so many producers exceed residue limits (and those are just the ones who get caught), I cannot in good conscience recommend eating meat that has had antibiotics used in its production unless you have independent assurance of the integrity of the producer from a third-party certifier. If you can be assured of the producer's integrity, I am confident that the residue limits established by the FDA and USDA are safe. But absent that verification, because of the short-term damage antibiotics can do to your intestinal flora and the long-term damage in breeding superbugs, I wouldn't touch them with a proverbial ten-foot pole, and neither should you.

Certain labels on meat are a solid assurance that no antibiotics were administered. These labels are: Organic, USDA Organic, No Antibiotics Administered, and Never Given Antibiotics.

Because many producers are unethical, they are willing to trade on the very legitimate concerns of their customers by labeling their products in a way that makes it seem that they were raised without antibiotics, when antibiotics were in fact used. Examples of such labels are: Natural, Antibiotic-Free, No Antibiotics Added, and No Antibiotic Residues. These are just fancy lies.

There are some third-party certifiers that independently verify that antibiotics have not been used (or that if they have been used, withdrawal periods and residue limits are observed with wider safety margins than the law requires). These include Global Animal Partnership, Food Alliance Certified, Animal Welfare Approved, American Grassfed Certified, Certified Human Raised and Handled, and Certified Naturally Grown.

## Microbiological Safety

Mass-produced meat is seriously dangerous stuff from a microbiological perspective. I look back at the occasions when I ate ground beef raw as a young adult, and I realize how lucky I am that I didn't accidentally die through sheer ignorance and stupidity. The prevalence of potentially lethal pathogens in the meat supply is absolutely terrifying.

In November 2012, Consumer Reports released the results of its examination of supermarket pork, revealing that 69 percent of the samples they took were contaminated with *Yersinia enterocolitica*, a bacteria that causes an extreme gastrointestinal illness. The majority of the *Yersinia* found was resistant to several important antibiotics. The tests found residues of the antibiotic ractopamine in 20 percent of the samples. Furthermore:

> Salmonella, staphylococcus aureus, or listeria monocytogenes, more well-known causes of foodborne illness, were found in 3 to 7 percent of samples. And 11 percent harbored enterococcus, which can indicate fecal contamination and can cause non-foodborne related infections such as urinary-tract infections. Most of the bacteria found were resistant to at least one of the tested antibiotic drugs. This is also worrisome because people infected by those bugs may need to take a stronger (and more expensive) antibiotic.[13]

Post-harvest interventions have improved the microbiological safety of beef overall,[14] but ground beef in particular has a poor record of safety, having caused 3,801 verified cases of food poisoning between 1998 and 2010. Chicken has been even worse, with 6,896 cases of food poisoning during the same period.[15]

For a bit of perspective, however, raw vegetables are the single largest cause of food-borne illness.[16] This is because the producers fail to observe common-sense precautions (as well as regulations)

---

[13] "Consumer Reports Investigation of Pork Products Finds Potentially Harmful Bacteria, Most of Which Show Resistance to Important Antibiotics," Consumer Reports Press Release, November 27, 2012.

[14] M. Koohmaraie *et al.*, "Post-Harvest Interventions to Reduce/Eliminate Pathogens in Beef," *Meat Science* 71, no. 1 (2005): 79–91,

[15] R. Rettner, "Top Meats That Can Make You Sick," *Live Science*, April 23, 2013.

[16] A. Besant, "Leafy Greens Leading Cause of Food-Borne Illness, CDC Says," *Global Post*, January 29, 2013.

about how long they should wait before harvesting produce after spreading raw manure on fields as a fertilizer.

Obviously, living life entails risks. You can't hide in a shell and be protected from everything and still live, but you can (and should) take the following precautions:

- Wash your hands, utensils, and cutting boards thoroughly, and then dry them with a paper towel.
- Wash produce. This entails scrubbing root vegetables with a brush, running more delicate produce under running water in a colander, discarding the outer leaves of greens, and blotting or rubbing dry with a paper towel.
- When you are working with raw meats and vegetables, avoid cross-contamination by using separate cutting boards and utensils. Wash your hands when switching tasks.
- Use a meat thermometer to assure meat is sufficiently cooked. The safe-tested guidelines issued by the USDA have recently changed.[17] Ground meats (including pork, beef, lamb, and veal) should reach an internal temperature of 160°F, poultry (parts or ground) should reach 165°F, whole cuts of pork, lamb, beef, and veal should reach 145°F, and seafood should reach 145°F. The meat needs to be allowed to rest for three minutes after the required temperature has been attained.
- Don't use foods past their expiration date; keep your refrigerator at 40°F or below and your freezer at 0°F or below.

Most of the microbiological contamination of meat comes as an inevitable result of dealing with a natural product. Animals make manure, and that manure has lots of nasty germs. They have manure on their feet and backsides, and sometimes they even roll in the stuff. When chickens are processed, for example, the carcass is scalded in order to facilitate removal of the feathers. This process mixes caked feces on the feet or rear of the animal with water and distributes it all over the skin.

---

[17] D. Van, "Cooking Meat? Check the New Recommended Temperatures," *Foodsafety.org*; available at www.foodsafety.gov/blog/meat_temperatures.html.

When I process chickens for meat, I take extreme care to do everything I can to prevent contamination and keep the meat safe by changing the scalding water for every bird, keeping everything hosed down and sterilized with bleach, removing entrails without getting feces on the bird, using rapid cooling, and so forth. But a single bird also takes me twenty minutes to process, which is unacceptable productivity for any sort of commercial operation that has to deal with market forces that keep retail prices low. The hard reality is that any mass-produced meat should be assumed to have fecal bacterial contamination of the surface, and ground meats should be assumed to have that contamination spread throughout. This, however, is not a problem so long as safe handling and cooking procedures are followed.

## If You're a Man, Eating Meat Makes You More Manly

Because humanity evolved to be human due to the inclusion of meat in the diet, one would naturally expect the benefits of a meat-based diet to be myriad—and they are.

One thing I have seen conspiracy theorists bemoan (and attribute to unknown actions by some conspiracy) is falling testosterone levels among men. Many men, whose testosterone levels are too low to support normal functioning turn to various (usually expensive) supplements or even testosterone supplementation. The low testosterone levels are also often attributed to environmental estrogens. While environmental estrogens (and soy) may well play a role, the two largest reasons for low testosterone levels are well within personal control: inadequate exercise and inadequate meat intake.

Exercise and meat go hand in hand in terms of male hormone levels. Each depends on the other, and they work together. Gobbling tons of steak while sitting on your butt won't help—you have to get moving. A study of male athletes demonstrated that when two diets of equal calories and equal total protein were compared, the diet whose protein was provided by meat resulted in significantly higher testosterone levels and significantly lower estrogen levels.[18] Another study in middle-aged men showed that low-fat diets decreased testosterone levels.[19] The fats in meat, particularly the saturated fats, also help to raise testosterone levels.[20]

When it comes to raising testosterone, not all forms of exercise are created equal. Resistance exercise raises testosterone, and it works even better with reduced rest periods between sets.[21] Sprinting likewise raises testosterone levels.[22] This means it is intensity and intervals rather than duration that makes the difference.

You can hardly turn on the television, open a magazine, or check your email without seeing ads for erectile dysfunction medications. Erectile dysfunction can have many causes. Low testosterone is one possible cause—curable with meat and exercise. Another cause, and a far more serious one, is damage to the inside of the blood vessels. Most of this damage is done by a high glycemic diet, and such a diet also inhibits your body's ability to make nitric oxide—the key catalyst that allows blood vessels to dilate to achieve an erection.[23] This is exacerbated by industrial vegetable oils that are high in polyunsaturated fatty acids, which create free radicals when cooked, and contain a surfeit of omega-6 fatty acids that inhibit the body's natural ability to fight inflammation.

---

[18] A. Raben *et al.*, "Serum Sex Hormones and Endurance Performance After a Lacto-Ovo Vegetarian and a Mixed Diet," *Medicine and Science in Sports and Exercise* 24, no. 11 (1992): 1290–97.

[19] C. Wang *et al.*, "Low-Fat High-Fiber Diet Decreased Serum and Urine Androgens in Men," *Journal of Clinical Endocrinology and Metabolism* 90, no. 6 (2005): 3550–59.

[20] J. S. Volek *et al.*, "Testosterone and Cortisol in Relationship to Dietary Nutrients and Resistance Exercise," *Journal of Applied Physiology* 82, no. 1 (1997): 49–54.

[21] R. Rahimi *et al.*, "Effects of Very Short Rest Periods on Hormonal Responses to Resistance Exercise in Men," *Journal of Strength and Conditioning Research* 24, no. 7 (2010): 1851–59.

[22] F. Derbré *et al.*, "Androgen Responses to Sprint Exercise in Young Men," *International Journal of Sports Medicine* 31, no. 5 (2010): 291–97.

[23] G. Rashid *et al.*, "Effect of Advanced Glycation End-Products on Gene Expression and Synthesis of TNF-Alpha and Endothelial Nitric Oxide Synthase by Endothelial Cells," *Kidney International* 66 (2004): 1099–106.

A diet high in omega-6 fatty acids provided by corn oil, soybean oil, and similar products stimulates the growth of prostate cancer cells.[24] Replacing animal fats with vegetable oil has certainly not done any favors for men.

Adopting a meat-based diet that discards high glycemic foods and industrial vegetable oil in favor of lean meats combined with the omega-3 found in fish will stop the progress of this problem and give the body a chance to heal.

## If You're a Woman, Eating Meat Makes you More Womanly

A diet high in proteins and low in carbohydrates dramatically improves a woman's fertility—by as much as 50 percent.[25] The lead researcher in the study, Jeffrey B. Russell, MD, at the Delaware Institute for Reproductive Medicine, reports some common sense based on his study: "Protein is essential for good quality embryos and better egg quality, it turns out." The high fat and low carbohydrate intake inherent in a meat-based diet has also been shown to raise estrogen levels.[26]

You may recall that in Chapter 7 I mentioned that overdoing exercise was problematic. Long-distance running/swimming/biking have all been tied to early onset of dementia and cognitive decline in women because they depress estrogen levels so that estrogen cannot protect the brain from the chronic inflammation.[27]

---

[24] M. Hughes-Fulford *et al.*, "Arachidonic Acid, an Omega-6 Fatty Acid, Induces Cytoplasmic Phospholipase A2 in Prostate Carcinoma Cells," *Carcinogenesis* 26, no. 9 (2005): 1520–26.

[25] American College of Obstetricians and Gynecologists, "High Protein, Low Carb Diets Greatly Improve Diets," May 6, 2003; available at www.acog.org.

[26] M. N. Woods *et al.*, "Hormone Levels During Dietary Changes in Premenopausal African-American Women," *Journal of the National Cancer Institute* 88, no. 19 (1966): 1369–74.

[27] C. Laino, "Strenuous Exercise Linked to Memory Loss," Web*MD*, available at www.webmd.com/fitness-exercise/news/20090715/strenuous-exercise-linked-to_memory-loss.

(Obviously, this is a name-your-poison sort of situation because lower hormone levels lead to chronic problems, such as dementia, and higher hormone levels are linked to hormonally sensitive cancers, such as breast cancer in women and prostate cancer in men, for people who are susceptible.)

You may not be surprised, given that evolution is driven by differentials in reproduction, to find that a host of studies correlate a woman's fertility with how attractive she is perceived to be by men. This applies to considerations of facial and vocal attractiveness within a woman's cycle,[28] but also to her general level of estrogen compared to other women. As one researcher described it, "there was a very strong and direct correlation between the level of each woman's oestrogen and how attractive, healthy and feminine they were found to be, showing that fertility is related to attractiveness."[29]

So the best action for a woman jilted by her boyfriend may not be a pint of ice cream. Not only will it make her acne flare up, but the high carbs will lower her natural estrogen levels. Instead, a steak (trimmed of visible fat), vegetables, and some moderate exercise are the ticket to replacing the ex-boyfriend with a better model in short order.

## Seafood

If you don't like seafood, you need to develop a taste for it. Modern meat raised in confinement operations has an adverse omega-6/omega-3 profile, and the omega-3s from vegetable sources are converted at a rate of only about 1 percent. So other than eggs, the only place you'll get the EPA and DHA you need to balance out the omega-6 fatty acids is fish. This is important for every system in your body.

---

[28] D. A. Puts *et al.*, "Women's Attractiveness Changes with Estradiol and Progesterone Across the Ovulatory Cycle," *Hormones and Behavior* 63, no, 1 (2013): 13–19.

[29] M. J. Law Smith *et al.* "Facial Appearance Is a Cue to Oestrogen Levels in Women," *Proceedings of the Royal Society B: Biological Sciences* 273 (January 2006): 135–40.

Wild seafood is better than farmed because the diet fed to many farm-raised fish reduces their omega-3 content to levels comparable to industrial meats. Mercury exists naturally in the environment, and all things ultimately find their way into the sea. Some of these things, such as mercury, tend to accumulate in tissues. The higher up the food chain a fish is, the more mercury concentrates in its meat. So larger fish, such as shark and swordfish, shouldn't be eaten more than once a week and should be avoided completely by pregnant women. It's best to concentrate on smaller species.

You may get sticker shock at the fish counter, but don't despair, because many species that are lower in price pack a solid nutritional punch, including mackerel, arctic char, cod, halibut, mussels, and oysters. Some of the discount chains also carry bags of frozen-at-sea salmon for a good price.

Canned seafood is also an excellent option, including salmon, mackerel, and sardines. Anchovies have a lot of DHA and go well on salads. "White albacore" tuna has about three times as much DHA as "chunk light" tuna. Because tuna, unlike other canned seafood, is cooked before canning, it isn't as high in EPA and DHA as other canned seafood.

Beware of seafood canned in oil as manufacturers most often use soybean oil, which contains enough omega-6 to wipe out the benefits of the omega-3 in the seafood. It pays to read the label. Another choice is smoked salmon, but be sure to read the package to make sure it doesn't contain preservatives—especially nitrites.

If you do freshwater fishing, bass, trout, catfish, and many other species are high in omega-3s and pretty much free in exchange for a relaxing day at the side of a pond, lake, or river.

## Eggs

Eggs are good for you. Particularly if you buy free-range or omega-3 enhanced eggs, they are a gold mine of nutriment. Eggs are high in anti-inflammatory omega-3s, vitamins E, B12, and lutein among other nutrients. Yes, they have fat. Yes, they have cholesterol. Yes the American Heart Association recommends no more than one egg a day. However, a recent meta-analysis following 263,938 people determined that egg consumption has precisely *zero* impact on coronary heart disease. The same analysis following 210,404 people found that increased egg consumption actually decreased the risk of hemorrhagic stroke.[30]

The only exception is in people with diabetes. Considering the material in the chapters on fats and carbohydrates, this makes sense. High levels of blood sugar cause the liver to produce small, highly reactive, and easily oxidized cholesterol, along with pumping out triglycerides like crazy. Normally, intake of saturated fat may raise overall cholesterol, but the type of cholesterol produced is actually cardioprotective or neutral. But if you add saturated fat to the diet of someone with poor blood sugar control, the result is increased cardiovascular risk.

If you follow a caveman diet, however, you are restricting your total daily glycemic load such that these sorts of issues don't affect you—so enjoy your eggs. I raise my own eggs and enjoy them over easy.

## Preserved Meats

Meats preserved via traditional methods such as drying (as jerky), pickling, canning, and freezing are perfectly healthy. The big thing you want to avoid is meat that contains preservatives, most especially sodium nitrite or potassium nitrite. (Some jerky does contain nitrites. Checking labels will help you avoid it.)

Meat products have a neutral to alkaline pH—usually 6.5 or higher. Anything with a pH higher than 4.8 can support the growth and multiplication of botulism bacteria, especially if it is packaged to exclude oxygen. Botulism bacteria produce a colorless and odorless toxin called botulinum that is an incredibly deadly neurotoxin. In fact, it is the most deadly poison known,[31] so even tiny amounts can cause lifelong aftereffects or death from paralysis.

---

[30] *BMJ* 346 (2013): e8539.

[31] S. S. Arnon *et al.*, "Botulinum Toxin as a Biological Weapon: Medical and Public Health Management," *Journal of the American Medical Association* 285, no. 8 (2001): 1059–70.

Mass-produced processed meats, such as bologna and sausage, are particularly susceptible to contamination with botulism, and to prevent killing their customers (which can be bad for business), manufacturers add sodium nitrite or potassium nitrite to inhibit the growth of botulism. Unfortunately, they avoid something that kills you quickly by adding a substance that kills you slowly.

The substances in tobacco smoke that give it a carcinogenic character are nitrosamines. The FDA has stated that there is *no* safe level of exposure. Nitrosamines can combine with DNA to create mutations. They don't always, but they *can.*

When sodium nitrite or potassium nitrate are united with a protein in an acidic environment such as the human stomach, they combine with the amino acids constituting the protein to make . . . nitrosamines. Though the FDA regulates the amount of nitrites that can be added to meats as a preservative in order to limit nitrosamine exposure to presumably safe levels, common sense indicates that eating meats preserved with nitrites is about as safe or unsafe as smoking. A diet high in vegetables and fruits can ameliorate the risk, but a reasonable person might ask if salami is really *so* good that it is worth the risk of eating it.

In the interest of fairness, I should state that most of the nitrites and nitrates (which turn into nitrites in the body) that we consume come naturally from vegetables.[32] There is, however, an important difference. Though nitrite is nitrite no matter the source, when nitrite is accompanied by vitamin C—which is abundant in vegetables—it doesn't turn into a form that reacts with amino acids to form nitrosamines. Instead, it passes through the stomach into the intestines intact, where intestinal bacteria turn it into nitric oxide, which helps to reduce blood pressure. This is why eating vegetables reduces your risk of high blood pressure.

I should also state, in further fairness, that the case against nitrites in meat is predominantly theoretical. That is, it is based on the fact that I can dump some potassium nitrite, protein, and

---

[32] L. Yoquinto, "The Truth About Nitrite in Lunch Meat," *Live Science*, December 30, 2011.

protease enzyme into diluted hydrochloric acid in a test tube, warm it gently over a Bunsen burner, and generate nitrosamines. There is no ironclad proof that the nitrites in salami end up making nitrosamines instead of nitric oxide in the intestines, because it is impossible to measure that in a living human being. Furthermore, the studies linking nitrite-preserved meats with colon cancer don't correct for other factors that could have a serious effect, such as consuming lectin-laden grains that strip the protective mucus from the intestinal lining.

Of course, another issue with processed meat is the use of fillers. A great many lunch meats contain wheat in various forms, and as I discussed in the chapter on grains, about 30 percent of people produce antibodies against the gluten in wheat, meaning it is eliciting an inflammatory response. With inflammation forming the basis of many chronic diseases, the fillers in processed meats are best avoided.

In general, you should consider the issue that perhaps it is unwise to consume something that is concocted in such a way that it can only be made safe enough that it won't kill you instantly by adding a veritable chemistry set in its production.

## The Bottom Line on Meat

Meat is good for you and is arguably the linchpin of our evolution into human beings. The best choice in meat is wild game, but that is obviously not an option for most people. Barring that, the next best choice is free-range, organic, and grass-fed meat. If these choices are too expensive, then the most important thing you want to avoid in meat is the added antibiotics, so look for labels identifying this fact. If you can't find meat without antibiotics, then go for poultry, which has a solid record of compliance with residual antibiotic levels a thousand times below the threshold of biological effect.

It is important that you have fish in your diet at least three times a week. Smaller fish are safer because they don't concentrate toxic metals to the same degree as larger fish. Canned fish is an especially good option if price is a problem, with mackerel, sardines, and salmon among the best choices and white albacore tuna as a distant fourth choice. Canned anchovies are also a good choice and go great in salads and dressings.

Legumes and grains are the primary alternatives to meat as a source of protein. These can certainly work in traditional environments where they are sprouted (to get rid of the antinutrients) and fermented (to diminish the lectins and hormonal disruptors), but in practice these techniques are too time consuming to be practical for most Americans on tight schedules. In addition, these do nothing to eliminate gluten and hormones that can be problematic. Though dairy can be a source of protein and fats, it comes with trade-offs, including increased risks of life-threatening auto-immune diseases. Almost any living thing has protein in it, and if you eat enough of it, you'll get enough protein. But that is usually combined with an inordinate amount of easily absorbed carbohydrate that will have other adverse effects.

Processed deli meats are often combined with gluten-containing fillers, and those that aren't are usually preserved with nitrites or nitrates that increase the risk of producing carcinogenic nitrosamines that are best avoided. (There are some brands of deli meat that contain no nitrites or nitrates.)

So meat is the safest source of protein for the human body. There is one qualifier: Mass-produced meat has serious issues with microbiological safety and therefore must be handled and cooked properly in order to avoid serious illness or even death.

And if all of that isn't convincing, meat will also make you a more manly man or a more womanly woman. So fire up the grill. Meat's back on the menu.

# Chapter 10
# The Modern Caveman Food Pyramid

The USDA has put together many food pyramids over the years, but due to pressure from a variety of quarters has finally abandoned the idea of a food pyramid with six to eleven servings of grain at its base. It has replaced the food pyramid with "My Plate," which shows a plate divided roughly in four parts—one part with grains, another with vegetables, the third with fruit, and the fourth with protein. Dairy is shown as a small image off to the side. Though this is clearly a vast improvement over the old pyramid, it still has serious deficiencies. I am going to cover the USDA guidelines first along with my critique and then present the modern caveman guidelines.

The USDA recommends one cup of fruit daily for children, and two cups daily for men and women. The USDA's "fruit" group includes fruit juices. Eating a piece of fruit is perfectly safe and healthy, but fruit juice, even "100 percent fruit juice," is no different from candy. Juice is made by squeezing the sugary liquid from a fruit and leaving the rest of the ingredients behind. If you have ever made juice with a juice machine, you learn quickly that it takes a *lot* of apples to make a glass of apple juice. Depending on the size of the apples, it could take a dozen. If you look at the label on practically any "100 percent juice" in the supermarket, you'll find its sugar content to be right in the same ballpark with soda and sometimes even higher. If you look at the nutrition label, you'll find that the stuff is nutritionally empty. At most, it has a tad of vitamin C, but even that was artificially added. A person would normally eat one or two apples but wouldn't normally eat a dozen. Fruit juices should be avoided because they keep the sugar while discarding other important nutrients.

The USDA recommends between one and a half and three cups of vegetables daily, depending on age and sex. By the time girls are eighteen, their recommendation matches that of women at two and a half cups, and when boys reach eighteen, their recommendation matches that of men at three cups. The major critique I have of this recommendation (other than that the quantity is insufficient) is that the USDA includes starchy roots in this category, such as potatoes and taro, along with grains, such as corn. These materials are, considering the way they are usually cooked, nutritionally vapid compared with green leafy vegetables, such as spinach, or other vegetables, such as tomatoes or cabbage. In addition, they are simple carbohydrates with a high glycemic load. Especially given that starchy grains are already included in a category, the last thing we need is people thinking they can fulfill their vegetable requirements with home fries.

The USDA specifies that half of all grains eaten should be "whole" grains—that is, have the germ intact. They specify a *minimum* of three "ounce equivalents" for women and four "ounce equivalents" for men but recommend six "ounce equivalents" for women and eight "ounce equivalents" for men. An "ounce equivalent" is a slice of bread, a cup of ready-to-eat cereal or half a cup of cooked pasta or rice. "Whole grains" are barely distinguishable from others in terms of glycemic load, and even neglecting the other adverse aspects, this still has grains forming the caloric backbone of someone's diet—a caloric backbone that has a high glycemic load.

The USDA classifies "meat, poultry, seafood, beans and peas, eggs, processed soy products, nuts, and seeds" as members of the protein group, specifying that women need five and a half "ounce equivalents" and men need six and a half "ounce equivalents" daily. The USDA states, "In general, 1 ounce of meat, poultry or fish, ¼ cup cooked beans, 1 egg, 1 tablespoon of peanut butter, or ½ ounce of nuts or seeds can be considered as 1 ounce equivalent from the Protein Foods Group." Though the USDA recommendations have improved by stating that we should eat at least eight ounces of seafood weekly, the emphasis on the interchangeability of legumes with meats is unwise, and the amount of protein specified is too low. Furthermore, most peanut butter—besides being a legume—is made with copious amounts of hydrogenated vegetable oil. Something made with hydrogenated vegetable oil doesn't belong in the human diet *at all.* It isn't food.

The USDA continues to push the doctrine of three cups of milk daily being necessary for men and women alike, forgetting that most people on the planet can't digest lactose. Nobody at the USDA is observant enough to notice that other mammals, such as elephants, bears, lions, and horses, develop impressive bone structures without any access to milk at all after weaning.

The current USDA guidelines push industrial vegetable oils high in omega-6 polyunsaturated fat in preference to saturated fat despite plentiful evidence that replacing saturated fats with poly-unsaturated fats is disastrous for cardiovascular health.

These guidelines are certainly an improvement over the pyramid they replaced, but they still leave high glycemic carbs as the basis of the diet, see legumes containing hormone analogs as a reasonable replacement for meat, replace the saturated fat from meats with high omega-6 polyunsaturated vegetable oils, and push dairy on a world that mostly cannot digest it. The USDA recommendations are high in lectins and antinutrients and continue to be based on high carbohydrate consumption. On the positive side, the USDA is emphasizing the importance of fruits and vegetables and has issued specific recommendations for fish.

Though the current USDA guidelines are not ideal from the perspective of the research I've presented in this book, they are nevertheless a step in the right direction and far better than the diet consumed by the average American. Even so, given the fact that the incidence of *all major chronic illnesses* and many others has *increased dramatically* since the government has got-ten involved in specifying diet, it might be worth considering that taking health advice from the same government that brought us

Project MK-Ultra,[1] the Tuskegee Experiment,[2] and COINTELPRO[3] might not be advisable. I'm not much of a conspiracy theorist, but one can never underestimate the results of incompetence and self-interest meeting political power. And the record of government dietary recommendations speaks for itself in terms of adverse outcomes.

## The Modern Caveman Dietary Guidelines

It is impossible to faithfully recreate the diet of ages past on anything approximating a reasonable budget, but we can come close enough to realize impressive health benefits using the foods available to us today.

A modern caveman diet can best be described as a stool with three legs forming its foundation and any extra materials on top. The first leg is protein, predominantly in the form of meat. The second leg is fat. Though much of that fat accompanies protein sources, it can also be supplied in the form of olive oil, coconut oil, avocados, etc. The third leg of the stool is composed of non-starchy vegetables and fruits. Once the stool has its three legs, it can hold up other things such as a small amount of carbohydrate from starchy roots, an occasional splurge on some flourless chocolate cake, or some aged cheese. But the key is that the foundation

---

[1] Project MKUltra was a secret federal program investigating mind control that lasted from 1953 to 1973. It involved the CIA, major pharmaceutical companies, dozens of colleges, and several hospitals. Many people were used as experimental subjects without their knowledge or consent, and in at least one known case, this resulted in death.

[2] The Tuskegee Experiment lasted from 1932 to 1972. Conducted by the U.S. Public Health Service under the guise of free health care, the experiment sought to follow rural African American men through the life cycle of syphilis rather than curing them, which could have easily been done.

[3] COINTELPRO was a secret federal program directed against political organizations deemed subversive that lasted from 1956 to 1971. Targets were discredited through psychological warfare, false media reports, and illegal force up to and including assassinations.

must be strong first, and the foundation is: meats, fats, and fruits and vegetables.

## Meats

Meat is key to the foundation of a sound human diet. Meat has a very high density of complete protein, fat, and nutrients. The protein triggers satiety, and the fat triggers peristalsis.

There is no set rule for protein consumption. Every person is different, and just in terms of feeling satiated so as to avoid the craving to chow down on pizza, different quantities of protein will be required.

The U.S. RDA for protein in a sedentary person is 0.36 g per pound of bodyweight. If you weigh 115 lbs, then you need 115 x 0.36 = 41 g of protein daily. If you weigh 190 lbs, then you need 190 x 0.36 = 68.4 g of protein daily. This is one recommendation that even contrary experts have found accurate over a period of decades. Though this recommendation is for sedentary people, it is more than sufficient for people who get moderate exercise so long as they also get enough fat. Going a little over or under—or even dramatically over or under—periodically won't hurt you. After all, sometimes a caveman had a successful hunting trip, and sometimes he didn't.

If you are an athlete, and I encourage you to be one because our hunter-gatherer ancestors were indeed athletes by modern standards, training is optimized with intake of between 0.46 g and 0.64 g of protein per pound of body weight.[4] If you are dieting to lose weight, increasing the amount of protein even further increases satiety and maximizes weight loss while helping to retain muscle.[5]

---

[4] S. M. Phillips and L. J. Van Loon, "Dietary Protein for Athletes: From Requirements to Optimum Adaptation," *Journal of Sports Science* 29, suppl. 1 (2011): S29–S38. Review.

[5] T. P. Wycherley *et al.*, "Effects of Energy-Restricted High-Protein, Low-Fat Compared with Standard-Protein, Low-Fat Diets: A Meta-Analysis of Randomized Controlled Trials," *American Journal of Clinical Nutrition* 96, no. 6 (2012): 1281–98.

This amounts to an average of 63 g of protein daily if you weight 115 lbs and 104 g of protein daily if you weigh 190 lbs.[6]

But this needs to be translated into something useful because nobody counts grams of protein. So here is a table to give you a rough idea of how much protein is in various foods.

| Food | Grams of Protein | Food | Grams of Protein |
|------|------------------|------|------------------|
| Canned tuna, 2 oz | 13 | Canned salmon, 2.5 oz | 13 |
| Turkey, 5 oz | 42 | Chicken breast, 5 oz | 35 |
| Lamb shoulder, 3 oz | 30 | Beef round, 3 oz | 30 |
| Beef chuck, 3 oz | 26 | Pork loin/ chops, 3 oz | 25 |
| Beef liver, 3 oz | 23 | Ground beef, 3 oz | 21 |

Translating this into practice, you should eat something containing protein at every meal, such as some salmon for breakfast,

---

[6] There is one other situation pertaining to protein that merits mention: cancer. Cancer cells are defective in many ways, and one of their defects is an inability to transition from a glucose-based metabolism (called the "mTOR pathway") to using ketone bodies. When cancer cells try to use ketone bodies from fat in their metabolism in place of glucose, they commit suicide (called "apoptosis") after accumulating too much free radical damage. In practice, carbohydrates in the diet feed both cancer cells and normal cells, but a diet in which carbohydrates are severely restricted and most calories come from fats will feed normal cells while starving cancer cells and causing them to commit suicide.

Though the mTOR pathway upon which cancer cells depend for survival is normally fueled with glucose, it can also be fueled by the amino acid glutamine. The glutamine comes from breaking down proteins. So when a ketogenic diet is used to combat cancer (as well as epilepsy and certain other diseases), protein is slightly restricted compared with the RDA. In this way, there is no excess glutamine available to fuel the cancer cells' metabolism. It is perfectly safe to have plenty of (natural) fat to balance out the lack of calories from other sources, and the fat will protect your body from breaking down its own proteins.

a pork chop at lunch, and some chicken for dinner. If you are already weight-proportionate, you don't have to go nuts on portion control. Just eat a reasonable serving of protein with each meal.

If you *are* overweight or obese, studies indicate that, at least during your period of weight loss, you'll benefit from eating levels of protein as much as double the U.S. RDA. Nobody ever became obese from gorging on salmon. The most likely culprits in that equation are simple sugars, high glycemic carbohydrates and industrial oils. As these aren't even on the modern caveman menu except in rare circumstances, you'll likely lose weight just by adopting a caveman diet. If, in faithfully following the diet you still don't lose weight, limit your protein intake to twice the RDA.

You should fit fish into your diet at least three times a week. (This is a minimum! More is better.) Other than that, eat eggs and whatever meats you would like, trimming any excess visible fat. Ideally, meats will be hunted. Most of us can't do that, so the next best is to go for grass-fed, free-range, or organic. If these options are unavailable or too expensive, the only really important thing is to avoid added antibiotics. If you are eating conventionally produced meats, then you should balance out their inflammatory omega-6 fats by increasing your fish consumption. Meats preserved with nitrites are probably best avoided except on rare occasions.

Eggs are perfectly okay for daily use. Pay no attention to the guy imposing artificial limits on the consumption of eggs based on their cholesterol content. The cholesterol in eggs is digested by most people rather than absorbed, and their omega-3 fats serve as anti-inflammatory compounds that reduce the risk of a host of ailments. Even if the cholesterol were absorbed, there is actually no link between cholesterol and heart disease per se. If you are concerned about heart disease, watch the triglycerides in your blood—and these are raised by simple carbs, such as those in grains or sugar. Two eggs are far better for your heart and health than two slices of toast or a "whole grain" muffin.

## Fats

Most of the fat in your diet will probably come from the meat you eat. Usually, just by eating meats, this will take care of itself. But if you are prone to eating exclusively low-fat meats, such as skinless chicken breast, tuna, or pork loin, your diet may be fat deficient. Fat deficiency can be a problem because the resulting caloric deficit will create uncomfortable levels of hunger that make it really hard to look away from donuts and cupcakes. Fat also helps to protect your muscles from being used as food by your body if you are in caloric deficit.

Additional fat in the diet can come from olive oil, walnut oil, avocado oil, coconut oil, and similar sources. Ideally, these will be virgin or extra-virgin with little or no heat used in processing. I happen to like buffalo, which is very low in fat, so I fry it in a bit of coconut oil so it doesn't stick. I eat a lot of salad and use olive oil to make the salad dressing. You can also use tallow (beef fat) or lard (pork fat) for frying. I use the grease collected from nitrite-free bacon for frying greens, and it's delicious!

The big things to avoid are the mass-produced industrial oils like soybean oil and corn oil especially, but also hydrogenated oils of all stripes along with canola and others. This can be hard to do, but I'll give you some tips for that later.

## Nonstarchy Vegetables and Fruits

Nonstarchy vegetables and fruits are the third leg of the stool. Nonstarchy vegetables, such as spinach and other greens, cabbage, broccoli, and onions among others, are crucial to your health and well-being. There is considerable evidence that eating your vegetables will make your life better in almost every way imaginable, and this is not surprising given the surfeit of vitamins, minerals, enzymes, and phytonutrients they provide.

Though it is well established that eating vegetables can help prevent nearly every chronic disease, the same doesn't apply to supplements. In fact, when it comes to supplements, quite the opposite is true except in a few cases. Studies of vitamin E (and vitamin E combined with selenium) demonstrate that the supplements increase the risk of prostate cancer.[7] Studies on beta-carotene supplements demonstrate a significantly increased risk of lung cancer.[8] Even vitamin C supplements work to protect cancer cells.[9]

You may be wondering how it can be that various studies can show reduced risks of cancer[10, 11, 12] from eating vegetables, as well as reduced risks of heart disease, stroke, macular degeneration, and a host of other ills, while supplements actually increase the risks. There are many reasons. In most cases, the industrially produced supplements are similar to, but not identical to, the compounds in plants, meaning they don't have identical effects in the body.

In other cases, the compound lacks context. By that I mean that the compound is being delivered in a pure pharmaceutical form that separates it from all of the other ingredients in the plant. The ingredients of a plant work together within your body. For example, the vitamin C in spinach makes the nitrites it contains into beneficial compounds for your blood vessels, whereas the nitrites taken by themselves would form carcinogenic nitrosamines.

---

[7] S. M. Lippman *et al.*, "Effect of Selenium and Vitamin E on Risk of Prostate Cancer and Other Cancers: The Selenium and Vitamin E Cancer Prevention Trial (SELECT)," *Journal of the American Medical Association* 301, no. 1 (2009): 39–51.

[8] "The Effect of Vitamin E and Beta Carotene on the Incidence of Lung Cancer and Other Cancers in Male Smokers, The Alpha-Tocopherol Beta Carotene Cancer Prevention Study Group," *New England Journal of Medicine* 330 (1994): 1029–35.

[9] American Association for Cancer Research, "Vitamin C Supplements may Reduce Benefit from Wide Range of Anticancer Drugs," Press Release, October 1, 2008.

[10] L. E. Voorrips *et al.*, "Vegetable and Fruit Consumption and Risks of Colon and Rectal Cancer in a Prospective Cohort Study: The Netherlands Cohort Study on Diet and Cancer," *American Journal of Epidemiology* 152, no. 11 (2000): 1081–92.

[11] M. G. Jain *et al.*, "Plant Foods, Antioxidants, and Prostate Cancer Risk: Findings from Case-Control Studies in Canada," *Nutrition and Cancer* 34, no. 2 (1999): 173–84.

[12] D. Feskanich *et al.*, Prospective Study of Fruit and Vegetable Consumption and Risk of Lung Cancer Among Men and Women," *Journal of the National Cancer Institute* 92, no. 22 (2000): 1812–23.

In addition to this, sometimes the supplements come in doses that vastly outstrip anything your body could possibly absorb normally, and thereby become a problem by reducing your body's ability to absorb or produce the nutrients normally. Also, whether or not something is healthy is often dependent on dosage. A small amount is healthy, but a large amount can be harmful. The bottom line is there is no shortcut: you must eat your vegetables.

How much is enough? Though it is pretty much impossible to eat too many vegetables under ordinary circumstances, at a bare minimum you need between four and six cups of vegetables daily. If you are eating lettuce or other green leafy vegetables, you need *two* cups for it to count as a cup because there is so much air space. This is your bare minimum. Outside of that consider there to be no limits. If you are overwhelmed by a desire to eat cherry tomatoes or okra until you pop, go right ahead.

When it comes to fruit, the bare minimum is two cups daily. If you are eating dried fruits, a quarter of a cup counts as a cup. Do, however, watch the glycemic load on dried fruits because some (such as raisins) are indistinguishable from a candy bar and others have added sugar. So limit dried fruits to a quarter of a cup daily.

In practice, then, you need to be eating two cups of vegetables and two-thirds of a cup of fruit at every meal.

If you are trying to lose weight and you have adopted caveman diet religiously but are having no success, then drop fruit from your diet. All of the nutrients available in fruits are also present in almost all vegetables, except that vegetables lack the simple sugars present in fruits.

## Everything Else on the Table

The base of the table is meat, healthy fats, fruits, and vegetables. These should be the core of your diet present at every meal because they provide your most important sustenance. Everything else is either optional (such as tree nuts) or something that should be included in your diet sparingly or in moderation if at all. I will cover this in the next chapter.

# Chapter 11
# Is It Caveman?

In my personal interactions encouraging people to adopt a caveman diet, I am usually confronted with a wall of questions regarding whether or not a particular food is or is not "caveman." The easy answer is this: If it existed or would have been reasonable for a caveman to produce it 15,000 years ago, then it is caveman. If not, then it isn't caveman.

This is a good rule of thumb for understanding the key issue, but it is also, for lack of a better word, a *religious* answer. We do not live 15,000 years ago; we live today. Cavemen didn't have Worcestershire sauce or brined dill pickles, but will you really die if you eat them? Cavemen didn't have vinegar for their salad dressing, but is vinegar really unhealthy just because they didn't have it?

When people are asking if something is "caveman," what they are really asking is: "Is it healthy, and to what degree can it be incorporated into my diet?"

There are, of course, people who are asking the question in a quest for legalistic loopholes. "You didn't mention that I couldn't eat manioc root, so I've decided that bread made with hyper-refined tapioca starch with a glycemic load even worse than white bread must be fine to eat three times daily." If someone is of that mindset, there is little I can do to help. I have, throughout this book, explained the principles and ideas, and these should suffice for the legally inclined if they are truly interested in improving their health rather than having a debate.

Earlier in the book, I defined two important concepts: caveman caution and caveman moderation. Everything that is not a natural meat, fat, vegetable, or fruit and that hasn't been prohibited as a grain or legume falls under a category to be used, if at all, with caution and/or moderation. That having been said, let's explore the larger categories.

## Starchy Roots

Starchy roots include starchy root crops that can be eaten if cooked and do not require extensive processing to be made safe. Examples of starchy roots include potatoes, sweet potatoes, parsnips, salsify, Jerusalem artichokes, yams, and beets. Not all roots are starchy. Carrots, onions, garlic, celeriac, and turnips are not starchy. Some starchy roots are deadly poison unless processed extensively. Manioc/tapioca is one example. By the time this is adequately processed it is nothing but sugar and nutritionally useless.

Starchy roots are high in either simple sugars (as is the case with beets) or starches that are readily converted into sugar, so they present a high glycemic load. That fact notwithstanding, starchy root crops often have high vitamin and mineral content, and they often contain unique ingredients that offset their risks. Beets, for example, contain compounds that even out blood sugar swings, and potatoes are high in B vitamins.

One benefit of starchy roots is that they can provide fast-acting carbohydrates that are free of the objectionable attributes of grains. These can come in handy during the one- or two-hour time frame following vigorous exercise that depletes the muscles' stores of glycogen. During this period, carbohydrates are converted directly to glycogen without impacting blood sugar at all. This helps your muscles recover and reduces muscular breakdown.

The key to keep in mind is that you should eat starchy roots in response to exercise you have just completed and *not* in anticipation of exercise you plan to do. You can, of course, eat them without benefit of exercise. Because they satiate easily, you are unlikely to overdo them as is common with grain-based and sugar-based carbohydrates. The only caveat is to avoid potatoes that have been fried in industrial vegetable oils.

Though it is a grain, I would include white rice in the same category as starchy roots because white rice has the antinutrients and lectins removed, so it is just a high glycemic starch.

## Vinegar

Though many purists of Paleo/Caveman/Primal diets argue that vinegar shouldn't be in the diet, because early modern humans wouldn't have had access to it, I don't think that is reason enough to eliminate it from the diet without further examination. Though early modern humans didn't typically eat grains or legumes, there are other reasons why they should not be consumed, and these are well documented.

Vinegar is diluted acetic acid made by acetic fermentation of alcohol. Like any other acid, it can be harmful if it is inordinately concentrated. The glacial acetic acid I have in my lab will burn a hole right through your skin and make a very painful burn. But most types of vinegar are in the 5 to 10 percent range, and there is absolutely no evidence that, used in moderation as a condiment, vinegar does any harm to people at all. In fact, there is abundant evidence that it is helpful.

There are many advocates of vinegar who argue that it cures cancer and so on. I have seen no credible evidence to substantiate these claims. However, there *is* very solid evidence that vinegar helps to increase satiety, reduce caloric intake, reduce the effective glycemic index of foods, and regulate blood sugar levels. By doing these things, vinegar would indirectly reduce the risk of metabolic syndrome, heart disease, and some cancers.

So vinegar absolutely belongs in the diet.

## Alcohol

In the chapter on carbohydrates, I covered the damage alcohol does to the skin. It is very dangerous stuff. Furthermore, some people have a genetic tendency to become addicted to alcohol, and this addiction can lower their quality of life, hurt people around them, and harm their health in a lot of ways. That having been said, there is evidence that moderate alcohol consumption can be beneficial for those who have genetic adaptations that make it safe for them to consume alcohol. Use extreme caution or avoid it altogether if there is a history of alcohol addiction in your family.

Beer is off the list because it is made from grain. Also, its nitrite level (which occurs naturally even if you make beer yourself) is high enough to make even a sausage salesman blush. Though beer is not as bad as the grains from which it is made, because the process of malting barley removes the antinutrients and the fermentation process takes care of many of the lectins, it can still present problems. A large portion of the population is either sensitive to gluten or could potentially develop a sensitivity. For people sensitive to gluten, there are often cross-reactions with similar (but not identical) proteins in other grains. Since inflammation sits at the base of practically all diseases of inflammation, it just makes no sense to drink beer.

Everything else is fair game. Though the form of alcohol for which we are likely best adapted is mead, hard cider, or wine, diluted distilled spirits are okay as well. Just keep in mind the necessity to use caveman moderation—no more than one serving three times weekly.

A few other cautions are in order. Never mix alcohol with an NSAID (non-steroidal anti-inflammatory drug), such as acetaminophen, ibuprofen, naproxen, or aspirin. If you do, serious liver damage could ensue. Also, many other medications come with warnings about taking with alcohol, and those warnings should be heeded.

## Salt

Salt is fine. I realize that the condemnation of salt is both knee-jerk and universal, but the cold, hard facts don't even come close to supporting such condemnations. Salt does not cause high blood pressure. Period. End of story, nothing more to see. The acceptance of the theory that salt causes high blood pressure is based on very flawed studies. The primary body of studies was performed on animals fed anywhere from ten to twenty times the amount of salt appropriate for the animals studied.[1]

---

[1] D. Brownstein, *Salt Your Way to Health*, 2d ed. (West Bloomfield, MI: Medical Alternatives Press, 2010).

The most often cited study supporting the theory is the INTERSALT study.[2] This was a study that encompassed fifty-two population centers. In forty-eight of the population centers, there was no correlation between sodium intake and high blood pressure, but in four population centers—encompassing tribes in Papua New Guinea, two Amazonian tribes in Brazil, and a tribe in Kenya—there seemed to be a correlation between low sodium intake and lower blood pressure. However, the study didn't correct for potential confounding variables, including a lack of obesity or alcohol consumption in those populations.

Basically, that is the full range of science supporting every doctor in the Western world insisting on the virtual elimination of salt from the diet. Meanwhile, other meta-analytical studies encompassing data from 1966 to 2001 show statistically insignificant effects on blood pressure.[3]

In addition, unnecessary salt restriction may in fact be hazardous. There is a large body of research indicating that salt restriction may increase one's risk of heart attacks,[4] increase the levels of insulin,[5] and retard the body's ability to remove excess levels of bromine.

The cause of high blood pressure is *insulin resistance*. Once you become insulin resistant due to insufficient exercise combined with excess carbohydrate intake, you will likely experience high blood pressure. This has been known (or at least strongly suspected) for more than twenty years. Dr. Reaven concluded an article that appeared in a 1991 edition of *Diabetes Care* as follows:

---

[2] P. Samler, *British Medical Journal* 312 (May 1996): 1249–53.

[3] N. A. Graudal, T. Hubeck-Graudal, and G. Jurgens, "Effects of Low Sodium Diet Versus High Sodium Diet on Blood Pressure, Renninm Aldosterone, Catecholamines, Cholesterols and Triglyceride," *The Cochrane Database of Systemic Reviews* 9, no. 11 (2011).

[4] M. Alderman, "Low Urinary Sodium Is Associated with Greater Risk of Myocardial Infarction Among Hypertensive Men," *Hypertension* 25 (1995): 1144–52.

[5] A. Rio *et al.*, "Metabolic Effects of Strict Salt Restriction in Essential Hypertensive Patients," *Journal of Internal Medicine* 233 (1993): 409–14.

There is evidence that insulin resistance and hyperinsulinemia occur commonly in patients with high blood pressure, and similar abnormalities have been described in several rodent models of hypertension. The challenge at this point is to define the potential mechanism and/or clinical importance, if any, of these changes. An argument has been developed that insulin resistance and hyperinsulinemia may play a role in both the etiology of hypertension and its ultimate clinical course. Given the unsatisfactory situation that exists in the effort to reduce the risk of CHD from high blood pressure, issues raised in this article deserve continued consideration.[6]

Later, other researchers comprehensively explained the precise mechanisms that link insulin resistance to high blood pressure.[7] The mechanisms are too complex to be explained thoroughly in a book like this, but if you are curious, I recommend looking up the cited articles. The gist is that elevated insulin levels impair the ability of kidney cells to excrete excess sodium. This, in turn, causes a buildup of sodium in the body and consequently retention of fluid within the blood, increasing its volume and hence its pressure.

Not everyone who is insulin resistant gets high blood pressure, but the overwhelming preponderance of people with high blood pressure are insulin resistant. I'm not a medical doctor, and even if I were, I don't know you personally, so I am not about to diagnose or treat a disease here.

But what I *am* going to tell you is that a medical degree is not a magical ticket to knowledge, and a lot of doctors blindly accept what constitutes conventional wisdom in their profession. Max Planck, the founder of quantum theory, wisely stated:

---

[6] G. Reaven, "Relationship Between Insulin Resistance and Hypertension," *Diabetes Care* 14, no. 11, suppl. 4 (1991).

[7] S. Horita *et al.*, "Insulin Resistance, Obesity, Hypertension, and Renal Sodium Transport," *International Journal of Hypertension* 2011, article ID 391762 (2011).

"A new scientific truth does not triumph by convincing its opponents and making them see the light, but rather because its opponents eventually die, and a new generation grows up that is familiar with it."

If you have insulin resistance or high blood pressure, you owe it to yourself to question authority because it is *your* health that is on the line.

But everyone else can and should eat salt. Salt is where your stomach gets the chlorine it needs to make hydrochloric acid. It helps to regulate and mediate practically every process in the body.

In terms of salt, I would personally recommend unrefined and minimally processed natural salts. Anything that is a pure crystalline white compound is a refined industrial product just as certainly as sugar. (Even if it is called "sea salt," if it is *white* it is *refined*.) Natural salts include products such as Celtic Sea Salt, Redmond's Salt, or Himalayan Salt, and they have distinctive coloration that may be gray, blue, or even pink. The primary benefit of these products over the cheap purified stuff is that they contain a plethora of trace minerals.

Refined salt contains two elements: sodium and chlorine. Unrefined salt contains eighty elements—all of the elements needed to support life. Our agricultural soils tend to be monocropped and overfarmed. Though the major macronutrients are restored in fertilizers, the micronutrients necessary for optimum human health are neglected. On my minifarm, I literally put (real) sea salt on my garden beds to provide those trace elements, but you can be certain that the commodity farmers aren't doing that. So switching from the industrial garbage to real salt can provide trace elements in your diet for optimal health.

A secondary benefit is flavor. Unrefined salt has a lively delicious flavor that leaves the taste of refined salt in the dust. If you have ever done a saltwater gargle, you know that refined salt has a distinctive chemical smell when mixed with warm water. If you do the same thing with unrefined salt, you'll notice a marked difference in the smell. The flavor difference is impressive, and you end up using less of it.

## Ketchup, Mustard, and Steak Sauce

Especially in America, these are absolute staples. The question is, can they be eaten in quantities suitable for a condiment without harm? The answer is yes.

Ketchup has a lot of sugar, about 4 g for a 1 tablespoon serving. Steak sauce has about 2 g for a 1 tablespoon serving. Mustard has no sugar. All three have added salt and vinegar. But just for context, an apple has 19 g of sugar. Every gram of sugar contains 4 calories. So a tablespoon of ketchup has 16 calories. If you eat 2,000 calories a day, then a tablespoon of ketchup is less than 1 percent of your caloric intake.

Though condiments you make yourself would be far superior nutritionally to anything you find in the supermarket,[8] the relatively small contribution of these condiments to the diet makes them, in my opinion, a nonissue. If they make your life and meals more enjoyable, have some!

## Mayonnaise and Salad Dressing

Most mayonnaise and salad dressings are made with soybean oil, and given the amount used and the high proportion of omega-6 polyunsaturated fats they contain, I cannot recommend their use in good conscience.

Salad dressings, such as Italian dressings that need to be shaken because the oil separates, can, however, be rehabilitated by replacing the lion's share of their soybean oil with olive oil. All you need to do is let them settle, then pour the soybean oil off the top carefully and add olive oil in its place. This will reduce the amount of soybean oil to a safe level. You can also make your own salad dressing using olive oil, vinegar, and seasonings.

---

[8] See the *Ball Blue Book of Canning and Preserving Recipes* for an excellent ketchup recipe, just replace the sugar with honey. See my book *The Mini Farming Guide to Vegetable Gardening* for everything you need to know about making your own mustard.

Traditional methods of making your own mayonnaise make it sound like a chore, but using modern equipment it takes less than five minutes, and the mayonnaise you make tastes great and will keep in the refrigerator for two weeks. The end result of using olive oil to make mayonnaise is called aioli, and it is available only at the finest restaurants unless you make it yourself.

## Soy Sauce and Worcestershire Sauce

Soy sauce can be made with or without wheat. The variety made with wheat should be avoided because there's a good chance you are sensitive to gluten. The variety that is made with "hydrolyzed soy protein" and maybe a bit of added salt or potassium sorbate is perfectly fine. This is because the fermentation process that turns soybeans into soy sauce destroys all the bad things in beans.

There is only one caveat. The amino acid that makes soy sauce a flavor enhancer and a universal additive for flavoring is glutamine. If you are on a ketogenic diet to treat cancer or epilepsy, you should avoid soy sauce because its glutamine content can fuel the mTOR metabolic pathway.

Worcestershire sauce often contains objectionable ingredients, such as molasses or high fructose corn syrup, but in small amounts. As with the case of ketchup or steak sauce, if a bit of Worcestershire sauce increases the quality of your life, there's no reason to avoid it.

## Concentrated Sugars

Concentrated sugars include table sugar, high fructose corn syrup, maple syrup, jams and jellies, molasses, agave nectar, honey, and similar items. None of these should be a mainstay or daily part of your diet.

Surely, I have been told, maple syrup must be a caveman food! Not so. If you tap a maple tree in the spring and drink the liquid flowing from it, it is barely sweet at all. Maple syrup is a result of evaporating most of the water until you have a concentrated sugar product. The same goes for agave nectar, molasses, and high fructose corn syrup. Table sugar is an industrial product. The only item on this list to which a caveman arguably had intermittent access is honey.

Fruit juice is also a concentrated sugar and should be avoided. Most juices (even "100 percent juice") contain as much sugar as Coca Cola or Pepsi. Some contain as much as 50 percent more! As fruit comes in nature, it provides checks and balances that allow you to gain nutrition without overeating. Apples are a great example. Apples have sugar, taste delicious, and provide a lot of fiber and vitamins. How many apples can you eat before you are sated and don't want any more apples? One? Two? Three, if you are starving? And if you eat those apples, they will come with a generous dose of fiber, vitamins, and minerals. But a twelve-ounce glass of apple juice will have virtually no vitamins, no minerals, and no fiber. It will, however, provide 39 g of sugar (just one gram less than Coke) and an impressive insulin spike.

With cave paintings depicting cavemen raiding a beehive, there is little doubt that humans have had access to honey for a long time. There are hundreds of varieties of stingless bees that make usable quantities of honey. Though these species don't live in temperate zones, they inhabit the areas around the equator on every continent. Because standard stinging honeybees are more economically effective at making honey, they have displaced the native stingless bees in many areas. Combined with the effects of development in rainforests, a number of species are at risk of extinction. Raising stingless bees for honey is a unique skill, and that skill is sadly dying out.

Though ancient people had the aid of the Greater Honeyguide (an African bird that will literally guide people to beehives), beehives aren't ubiquitous, and many bees do in fact sting, so access to honey would not have been a daily thing. So use honey sparingly and only intermittently. Caveman moderation (no more than thrice weekly!) is warranted. I use honey to make caveman chocolate cake every couple of weeks. Incidentally, you want only raw, unpasteurized honey, because in its raw form honey contains a lot of beneficial enzymes and proteins.

What is a caveman chocolate cake? Two cups of almond flour, ¼ cup of cocoa powder, ¾ cup of honey, four eggs, 1 teaspoon vanilla, ¼ teaspoon cinnamon, 1 teaspoon aluminum-free baking powder, and enough water to make it the right consistency for cake. Pour into a greased cake pan and bake at 350°F until a toothpick comes out clean (about twenty-five minutes, depending on the pan). Who says modern cavemen can't live the good life? This sort of thing is a rare treat rather than a daily staple, but it is definitely delicious.

There is one very important warning for honey: do *not* give it to infants. The digestive tract of infants doesn't have a fully functioning ecosystem of gut flora. As a result, botulism spores in honey that would be harmless for an adult can take root in the anaerobic environment of a baby's intestines, make botulinum toxin, and kill the baby.

## Milk Products

Many people can't digest lactose, so they obviously can't drink milk or eat yogurt. Most hard and aged cheeses lack lactose, so they can be eaten readily. There are, however, trade-offs to eating milk products. All milk products contain hormones that can encourage acne. When provided to children, there is evidence that milk may lay the groundwork for the later development of type 1 diabetes or multiple sclerosis. The process of lactose utilization can impair a woman's fertility. Low fat milk products in particular generate an insulin response far in excess of what would be expected based strictly on sugar content.

On the other hand, full-fat dairy products such as cheeses and butter have been demonstrated to reduce the risk of heart disease.

Children, in my opinion, should be allowed no dairy products except butter until they are teens, because butter lacks milk proteins. Anyone with acne should avoid all dairy, including butter. Everyone else, or at least those who like it, should consume dairy (primarily in the form of butter and cheese) with caveman moderation—no more than three servings weekly.

## Chocolate

Chocolate is definitely a refined product, though nowhere near as refined as industrial oils. Cocoa beans arriving at the factory are either made directly into chocolate liquor by grinding or separated into cocoa powder and cocoa butter. The cocoa powder may be treated with a light alkali.

Chocolate and cocoa powder contain antioxidants and flavanoids that impart valuable health benefits. Benefits include antiaging, [9] lowered blood pressure, [10] improved vascular function,[11] and reduced cardiovascular disease.[12] There is also evidence they improve learning and memory[13] while reducing the risk of death from all causes.[14] There is little doubt that, in and of itself, chocolate (meaning chocolate liquor from liquefied beans or cocoa powder) is a beneficial dietary addition. The key question is, what else is it mixed with?

---

[9] S. Mehta, "Pharmacognosy and Health Benefits of Chocolate," *PharmaXChange*, July 2013; available at http://pharmaxchange. info/press/2013/07/pharmacognosy-and-health-benefits-of-cocoa-seeds-chocolate/.

[10] D. Taubert, R. Roesen, and E. Schömig, "Effect of Cocoa and Tea Intake on Blood Pressure: A Meta-Analysis," *Archives of Internal Medicine* 167, no. 7 (2007): 626–34.

[11] H. Schroeter *et al.*, "(-)-Epicatechin Mediates Beneficial Effects of Flavanol-Rich Cocoa on Vascular Function in Humans," *Proceedings of the National Academy of Sciences* 103, no. 4 (2006): 1024–29.

[12] E. Ding *et al.*, "Chocolate and Prevention of Cardiovascular Disease: A Systematic Review," *Nutrition & Metabolism* 3, no. 2 (2006).

[13] V. Bayard *et al.*, "Does Flavanol Intake Influence Mortality from Nitric Oxide-Dependent Processes? Ischemic Heart Disease, Stroke, Diabetes Mellitus, and Cancer in Panama," *International Journal of Medical Sciences* 4, no. 1 (2007): 53–58.

[14] B. Buijsse *et al.*, "Cocoa Intake, Blood Pressure, and Cardiovascular Mortality: The Zutphen Elderly Study," *Archives of Internal Medicine* 166, no. 4 (2006): 411–17.

A lot of the chocolate candy you can get at the store is unsuitable for human consumption and contains a variety of ingredients that will negate any benefits from the chocolate. As one example, an expensive premium brand that I found at the grocery store contains hydrogenated soybean oil, high fructose corn syrup, and added lactose. It contains 24 g—about 100 calories worth—of sugar for a very modest serving. This is trash and nonfood. However, I found another premium brand in the organic section that contained no objectionable ingredients except 15 g of sugar per twelve pieces. That's actually not horrible, assuming the rest of your diet is solid, and you can always choose to eat just six pieces.

So if you love chocolate, please have some! Just be careful about what else has been added. In general, you'll be better off sticking to organic brands. Another option is to take it as hot chocolate. To make hot chocolate, mix one tablespoon of honey, a quarter of a teaspoon of vanilla, and one heaping teaspoon of cocoa powder with enough hot water to make six to eight ounces.

My grandfather was quite vigorous into late old age. I remember fixing fences with him in his eighties, and seeing him throw around 96 lbs bags of fertilizer like they were nothing. Though certainly his diet rich in free-range meats and home-grown vegetables combined with vigorous daily exercise had something to do with it, he always had a cup of cocoa in the morning to start his day. He was a tough guy though, because if I remember correctly, he used only a touch of sugar.

## Coffee and Tea

I think if the coffee and tea supplies were shut down, America would grind to a halt. Though I am sure many people throughout the world likewise enjoy these beverages, it is only in America where I have had to come to a complete stop in the middle of a major thoroughfare due to backups of people going through the drive-through of a coffee shop.

Coffee has benefits and detriments. Coffee has a lot of caffeine, which is addictive, and caffeine withdrawal can result in blinding headaches. So drinking coffee habitually can create an expensive dependency. Some of the otherwise beneficial compounds in coffee can bind to iron, so it isn't absorbed from the intestinal tract. Very high levels of consumption—four or more cups daily—can increase markers of inflammation,[15] which of course increases the risks of most chronic diseases. Because caffeine is a stimulant (and coffee also contains compounds that increase the release of adrenaline), it can be bad news for people suffering from anxiety disorders and panic attacks. Such disorders have become very common, and folks who have them should avoid coffee.

On the other hand, when consumed in moderation (four or fewer cups daily), coffee reduces the risk of developing type 2 diabetes,[16] liver cancer,[17] aggressive prostate cancer, cavities, dementia,[18] and death from heart disease.[19]

One of the major problems with coffee in the modern world is its packaging. Some of the premium coffee drinks at major chains pack a whopping 650-calorie high-sugar punch that kills waist-lines. If you weigh the risks and benefits of coffee against your own situation and opt to drink coffee, I would encourage you to drink it black with nothing added.

Tea, though originating from a very different plant, also contains caffeine, though generally not as much as coffee. A twelve

---

[15] A. Zampelas *et al.*, "Associations Between Coffee Consumption and Inflammatory Markers in Healthy Persons: The ATTICA Study," *American Journal of Clinical Nutrition* 80, no. 4 (2004): 862–67.

[16] S. N. Bhupathiraju *et al.*, "Caffeinated and Caffeine-Free Beverages and Risk of Type 2 Diabetes," *American Journal of Clinical Nutrition* 97, no. 1 (2012): 155–66.

[17] M. Inoue *et al.*, "Influence of Coffee Drinking on Subsequent Risk of Hepatocellular Carcinoma: A Prospective Study in Japan," *Journal of the National Cancer Institute* 97, no. 4 (2005): 293–300.

[18] "Midlife Coffee and Tea Drinking May Protect Against Late-Life Dementia," *Science Daily*, January 15, 2009; available at www.sciencedaily. com/releases/2009/01/090114200005.htm.

[19] A. Koizumi *et al.*, "Coffee, Green Tea, Black Tea and Oolong Tea Consumption and Risk of Mortality from Cardiovascular Disease in Japanese Men and Women," *Journal of Epidemiology and Community Health* 65 (2011): 230–40.

ounce cup of coffee contains between 100 mg and 160 mg of caffeine, whereas green or black tea contains anywhere from 40 mg to 120 mg for a similar quantity, depending on how it is brewed. So tea can have the same addictive quality as coffee. Though there are many forms of tea, most can be described as white, green, or black.

White tea is minimally processed. The buds and leaves are allowed to wither naturally, then the leaves are dried and shipped. Because of this minimal processing, white tea has the highest levels of antioxidants and other beneficial compounds of any type of tea. White tea is an antiaging panacea in that along with the usual health benefits of tea, it contains compounds that inhibit the breakdown of collagen and elastin in the skin.[20]

Green tea is gathered while still green and is allowed to wither. Then it is steamed (to stop detrimental enzymes), rolled, dried, and shipped. The compounds in green (but also white) tea reduce the risk of heart disease[21] and have shown promise as anti-inflammatory aid and in inhibiting cancer.[22]

Though most health research has focused on green tea, studies indicate that black tea reduces the risk of stroke[23] and reduces cardiovascular disease risk by reversing endothelial dysfunction.[24] Unlike white and green teas, black tea undergoes a full fermentation process that results in a wide array of complex flavors.

---

[20] T. S. A. Thring, P. Hili, and D. P. Naughton, "Anti-Collagenase, Anti-Elastase and Anti-Oxidant Activities of Extracts from 21 Plants," *BMC Complementary and Alternative Medicine* 9, no. 27 (2009).

[21] M. W. Huff and E. E. Mulvihill, "Antiatherogenic Properties of Flavonoids: Implications for Cardiovascular Health," *Canadian Journal of Cardiology* 26 (2010): 17A–21A.

[22] C. S. Yang and X. Wang, "Green Tea and Cancer Prevention," *Nutrition and Cancer* 62, no. 7 (2010): 931–37.

[23] S. C. Larsson, J. Virtamo, and A. Wolk, "Black Tea Consumption and Risk of Stroke in Women and Men," *Annals of Epidemiology* 23, no. 3 (2013): 157–60.

[24] S. J. Duffy *et al.*, "Short- and Long-term Black Tea Consumption Reverses Endothelial Dysfunction in Patients with Coronary Artery Disease," *Circulation* 104, no. 2 (2001): 151–56.

The bottom line on tea is that it is good for you overall but has the same contraindications as caffeine generally: It can be mildly addictive and can exacerbate problems with anxiety and panic attacks.

## Artificial Sweeteners

The general idea of artificial sweeteners is that they allow people to eat things that taste as though they contained sugar without having to pay the caloric price. They are most commonly added to soft drinks, though they can also be found in yogurts and other foods.

There is not, at this time, substantive research indicating that artificial sweeteners are harmful. There are some interesting studies indicating that drinking diet soda may make you fat, but if you look carefully at these studies, they are of an observational nature where other factors cannot be controlled—so they are suggestive at best and by no means definitive. Meanwhile, their use is endorsed by an impressive array of medical organizations.

Are they caveman? Strictly speaking, no. They are clearly industrial chemicals that are a very new addition to the human diet. As such, their potential harms are unknown.

It is worth recalling that trans fats were introduced into the food supply starting in the early 1900s and that even though many researchers expressed concern about their impact on human health as early as the 1950s, it wasn't until the 1990s that they were acknowledged as being dangerous. An industrial chemical can be added to our food supply, widely promoted as healthy, and consumed by millions and indirectly cause millions of early deaths for nearly 100 years before anyone seriously questions it.

As another example, aspirin has been used for over a century, and only now has it been discovered as a substantial risk factor for age-related macular degeneration.[25] It took a century to discover

---

[25] G. Liew "The Association of Aspirin Use with Age-Related Macular Degeneration." *Journal of the American Medical Association Internal Medicine* 173, no. 4 (2013): 258–64.

that a widely used and ubiquitous product raises the risks of macular degeneration by a very substantial 264 percent.

Furthermore, the fact that some recognized medical body endorses something doesn't really mean much. In spite of the fact that there was credible scientific evidence that tobacco was a substantial risk factor for various diseases starting at least from the 1930s,[26, 27] the American Medical Association allowed doctor endorsement of tobacco up through the 1950s and even derived millions of dollars in advertising revenue from publishing tobacco ads in the prestigious *Journal of the American Medical Association.*[28]

Even today, experts pretend that they were utterly ignorant of the potential hazards of tobacco until the 1950s. But I have a number of medical books in my possession from the 1800s, and many of them note associations between tobacco and serious illnesses. Even King James noted in 1604 that tobacco use was "[a] custome lothsome to the eye, hatefull to the Nose, harmefull to the braine, dangerous to the Lungs, and in the blacke stinking fume thereof, neerest resembling the horrible Stigian smoke of the pit that is bottomelesse." So the dangers were known for *centuries*.

No matter what oaths they take or what they claim as organizational objectives, most organizations have as their first imperative their own promotion and survival. It is in their best interest for you to surrender independent thought and rely solely on them. But is it in *your* best interest?

Common sense tells you that anything produced using hazardous materials in a facility requiring comprehensive personal protective equipment for workers is not *food* and that placing

---

[26] A. H. Roffo, "Krebserzeugende Tabakwirkung [Carcingogenic Effects of Tobacco]" (1940).

[27] R. N. Proctor, "The Anti-Tobacco Campaign of the Nazis: A Little Known Aspect of Public Health in Germany, 1933–45," *British Medical Journal* 313 (December 1996): 1450–53.

[28] B. Weeks, "Dateline: 1950 AMA Endorsed Tobacco => $9 Million," Weeks*MD*, May 24, 2008; available at http://weeksmd.com/2008/05/dateline-1950-ama-endorsed-tobacco-9-million/.

nonfood in one's mouth carries at least the *risk* of being hazard-ous. It might be 100 years before any hazards are finally brought to light.

Furthermore, products containing artificial sweeteners provide no real benefits to balance their potential harm. Diet soda would be harmful to your teeth anyway, as it usually contains phosphoric acid. Brominated vegetable oil is used in many soft drinks and sports drinks, and its excess consumption can lead to bromism—neurological damage from bromine toxicity.

At first blush, you'd expect that folks who use products con-taining artificial sweeteners would at least consume fewer calories overall so they would lose weight, but this doesn't seem to be the case. In fact, there seems to be no difference, indicating that what-ever calories someone fails to derive from a diet product are con-sumed elsewhere.[29] So you have potential risks without benefits.

So I advise caveman caution in approaching these chemicals. There has been enough testing that I doubt incidental quantities in sugarless gum and the like are particularly hazardous, but I recommend against having them as a substantial part of your diet by drinking two liters of diet soda daily, etc. If you are addicted to the caffeine in diet sodas, I encourage you to switch to coffee or tea.

## Yes, Cooking Is Caveman!

There's a wiseacre in every crowd. Somewhere out there, I can hear somebody muttering that in order to eat in conformance with our evolution, we have to stop cooking our food. No doubt, there is benefit to eating certain foods raw because their enzymes and nutritive qualities are intact. However, there is another side to this issue that few suspect.

I have mentioned in previous chapters that scientists believe it was our consumption of meat (and especially animal fat) that facil-

---

[29] S. Swithers, "Artificial Sweeteners Produce the Counterintuitive Effect of Inducing Metabolic Derangements," *Trends in Endocrinology and Metabolism* 24, no. 9 (2013): 1–11.

itated our comparatively large brain volume. But that is not the whole story. The rest of the story is a matter of how many calories can be consumed in a day from raw foods. In order to support a brain the size of a modern human (which, incidentally, is smaller and has fewer neurons than our preagricultural ancestors) on a raw food diet, we'd have to eat continuously for more than nine hours a day. It is only through cooking—predominantly of meat and tubers—that humans were able to get enough calories in a day to support a brain that consumes 20 percent of our caloric intake.[30]

The key changes that made us human then are twofold. First was the addition of meat (and especially DHA and EPA from meat), which gave our bodies the raw material from which brain can be formed. Next came cooking, which makes food more easily digested so it has a greater net caloric contribution and its nutrients are more available. Between the two innovations, we are smart enough to send our species to the Moon and engage in elaborate charades of self-deception.

---

[30] "Raw Food Not Enough to Feed Big Brains," *Science*, October 22, 2012; available at http://news.sciencemag.org/evolution/2012/10/raw-food-not-enough-feed-big-brains.

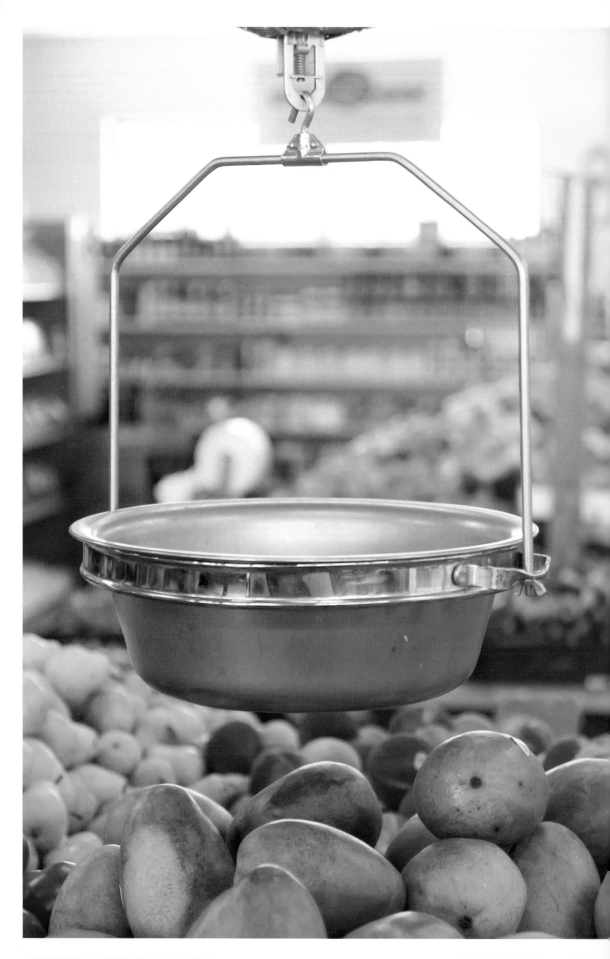

# Chapter 12
# Supermarket Checklists

One of the best aspects of a caveman diet is grocery shopping because you no longer have to dutifully slog down every aisle in the grocery store in case you forgot something. Nearly every aisle in the grocery store containing stuff in boxes and bags can be ignored. Pasta? Nope. Crackers? Nope. Juice? Nope. Ninety percent of your shopping is done around the outside perimeter of the store where you get fresh fruits and vegetables, meat, and eggs. You may make side trips down the freezer aisle for frozen vegetables, the baking aisle for spices, or the condiment aisle for some olive oil, but most of your shopping will be along the outside perimeter of the store where there is lots of room.

If you don't enjoy food shopping, you'll find that one of the best aspects of caveman diet is it easily cuts your time at the super-market in half. If you have joined the rising numbers of people growing at least a portion of their own food, then your visit to the supermarket will be even shorter.

In spite of the previous chapters, there may still be some questions, so I'll go through the supermarket sections to highlight important points.

## Produce Section

All fruits and vegetables are on the menu except that dried fruits should just be an occasional treat. Prefer organic fruits and vegetables if they are available and affordable, but if they aren't, don't worry, because all the studies on the wonders of fruits and vegetables were done on conventional (nonorganic) vegetables.

If you want to make sauces and need a thickener, there are two approaches I recommend. The first is to put dehydrated mushrooms into a food processor and reduce them to powder—they make an excellent thickener. The second is okra, which releases a thickener when cooked.

Make sure to get green leafy vegetables and materials for salads because you should be eating one salad daily. When I make salad, I usually make several at once and put them in the fridge for the next few days.

## Fresh Deli and Seafood Counter

The deli should be ignored. Most of the meats are preserved and processed, and even simple items like potato salad are likely adulterated with garbage, such as soybean oil in the mayonnaise.

Though it is expensive, smoked salmon portions (assuming they haven't been preserved with nitrites—some brands are, and some aren't) make a very convenient on-the-go food. Go for the smaller and less expensive fish for lower levels of mercury, and prefer wild over farm-raised fish for higher omega-3 content. Eschew tartar sauce, and learn to make your own. Cocktail sauce is fine.

If you can't find reasonably priced fresh fish, look in the frozen section. If you still can't find reasonably priced fish, go to the end of the canned goods aisle for canned fish. Make sure it is in either water or olive oil. Sardines, salmon, mackerel, herring, tuna, and more are available.

## Egg and Dairy Section

Eggs are great and can be eaten in a dozen creative ways. Prefer cage-free, organic, and high omega-3 varieties. They are more expensive but often have substantially more nutrients.

Forget any and all low-fat milk products, and avoid yogurt with sugar or artificial sweetener. If, after reading the chapter on dairy, you decide to eat dairy products, go for hard and aged cheeses if you are lactose intolerant. Absolutely avoid any and all so-called cheese food products. These may be good for caulking your bathtub but are otherwise unfit for human consumption. Butter is far more healthy than any industrial vegetable oil, but avoid it if you have intractable problems with acne.

## Bacon, Ham, Sausage, and Packaged Cold Cuts Section

Most of this stuff is infused with at least one objectionable additive and usually more. However, if you look carefully, in most supermarkets you'll find at least one uncured bacon variety available. Uncured ham is usually available only seasonally. Unless you are at one of the expensive natural food stores, cold cuts without additives are hard to find, but they are available at some grocery stores.

Sausage without additives is more likely to be found in the natural meats section than in the usual sausage section. Also, check the frozen foods section as some of the prepackaged sausage brands are free of additives. Be careful to read the ingredients as some sausages (especially those that are maple flavored) have enough sugar to sink a battleship.

## Canned Goods and Soups

It is difficult to find canned soup that has no grains or added sugars. You would naturally expect soups with names like "Chicken and Vegetables" to be devoid of grain, but usually wheat is added as a thickener. Even in the organic section, other than plain broth, it is really hard if not impossible to find grain-free soups. If you want them, you'll have to make them yourself.

Canned vegetables are not as good as frozen or fresh, but they are still a viable option especially if you are on a tight budget. Even without a tight budget, small cans of spinach, sauerkraut, and asparagus can come in handy.

You'll also find canned fruits and applesauce. Unsweetened applesauce is fine, but most canned fruits are sweeter than politicians on Election Day and should be avoided.

Canned seafood is fine provided it is canned in water or olive oil. Canned salmon, mackerel, sardines, anchovies, and more are available and can provide the DHA and EPA omega-3 fatty acids you need.

## Condiment Section

You'll usually find vegetable oils here. All you want is olive oil, walnut oil, coconut oil, high-oleic sunflower oil, and palm kernel oil. Flax oil is okay if you can stand it, but it must be refrigerated once opened to keep it from oxidizing. Ignore all the others unless you want to use them to make biodiesel or as massage oils.

Because of the high amount of omega-6 oils, most mayonnaise and salad dressing can be ignored. For those varieties that have oil floating on top, you can pour it off and substitute olive oil, but one of the reasons manufacturers don't use olive oil is because it solidifies in the refrigerator. That's not really a big deal—just take it out of the refrigerator a bit before the meal so it has time to liquefy before use.

Ketchup, mustard, gluten-free soy sauce, steak sauce, Worcestershire sauce, and similar condiments are fine when used as condiments. Organic versions tend to be more healthy and lower in sugar, but the quantities normally used are so small compared with the rest of the diet that you can get by with small amounts of regular condiments just fine.

Olives are usually unadulterated, but you should read the labels on pickles and relishes carefully as they often contain artificial colors that are best avoided. Ingredients such as lactic acid are perfectly fine. (Lactic acid naturally occurs in the human body.)

## Frozen Foods

Obviously, TV dinners are out of the question, along with prepared entrées and frozen pizza. However, raw ingredients such as frozen vegetables, fruits, and meats are fair game. Many times, the quality and nutritional value of frozen products are better than those of fresh products from the produce section. Frozen vegetables are good to have around for recipes as well as vegetable courses.

Frozen juice is a bad idea, along with ice cream, ice milk, frozen yogurt, and so forth.

## Cookies, Crackers, Chips, and Snacks

There is usually nothing to eat in these sections. The cookies and crackers overwhelmingly contain wheat, the chips are usually fried in industrial oils high in omega-6, and the snacks are full of five-syllable chemicals.

About the only two things of interest you'll find here are nuts and popcorn. Nuts are fine in moderation—just read to see what oils were used in their manufacture. If you can't find any suitable nuts, head over to the baking section where you can find packaged shelled nuts that haven't had oils used to make them. Nuts are totally caveman, but skip peanuts because they are actually legumes rather than nuts.

Strictly speaking, popcorn is not on the menu. However, as a rare indulgence while watching a movie, it isn't the end of the world. Popcorn is not genetically modified yet. Though it has a high glycemic index, it has a very low glycemic load because it is mostly air. A lot of microwave varieties have strange chemicals, so I recommend making it from whole popcorn using coconut oil. Sprinkle with some unrefined sea salt, and top with a bit of melted butter if you are inclined.

In health food stores you may find some more healthful snacks, including seaweed and various vegetables fried in either olive or avocado oil. These are fine so long as you take into account their carbohydrate content by reading the nutrition label.

## Dry Goods and Baking Sections

All forms of pasta and noodles are off the menu, as well as wheat, corn, barley, rye, spelt, and other grain-based or legume-based flours. Cereals are likewise off the menu. As discussed in prior chapters, grains are not a healthful addition to the diet. Even if grains weren't intrinsically unhealthy due to lectins, antinutrients, and lectin, processed cereals and pastas would be a poor choice for sustenance.

Just look at the ingredients on the side of practically any box of cereal. In most cases it is at least a two-inch column in six-point type. The reason is that the processing strips away practically all useful vitamins and minerals that occur naturally, and these are then added back in the form of artificial compounds. (There is no evidence that this "enrichment" does anything positive for human health.) Then look up their glycemic load for the amount of cereal you actually use rather than the minuscule serving size they list on the box.

This is nonfood. In fact, the closest analog I can find to this junk is dry pet foods. And you know what? We probably shouldn't be giving pets the stuff we give them either. But that's an exploration for another day.

The two flours you'll find in a well-stocked baking section that are worth getting are coconut flour and almond meal. Both are useful for making caveman-friendly equivalents of baked goods—the crust for an apple pie, for example. You can also pick up some honey—preferably raw honey. (This may be in the natural foods section rather than the baking section.)

Along with this, the whole array of herbs and spices is available to you. You should read the sides of any premixed spices because a lot of them use cornstarch and similar items as fillers. What you want is the plain spice.

When it comes to salt, if it is available, you should pick an unrefined variety for the micronutrients it can add to your diet. If you can't get unrefined salt, then the refined stuff is fine as are the spice mixes intended to emulate salt.

Products in the baking section containing potassium chloride as a salt substitute should be avoided, in my opinion, unless specifically recommended by a competent professional. Numerous people have wound up in the hospital due to interactions between these products and various medications. Unless you have a very specific reason for using them, they are best left on the shelf.

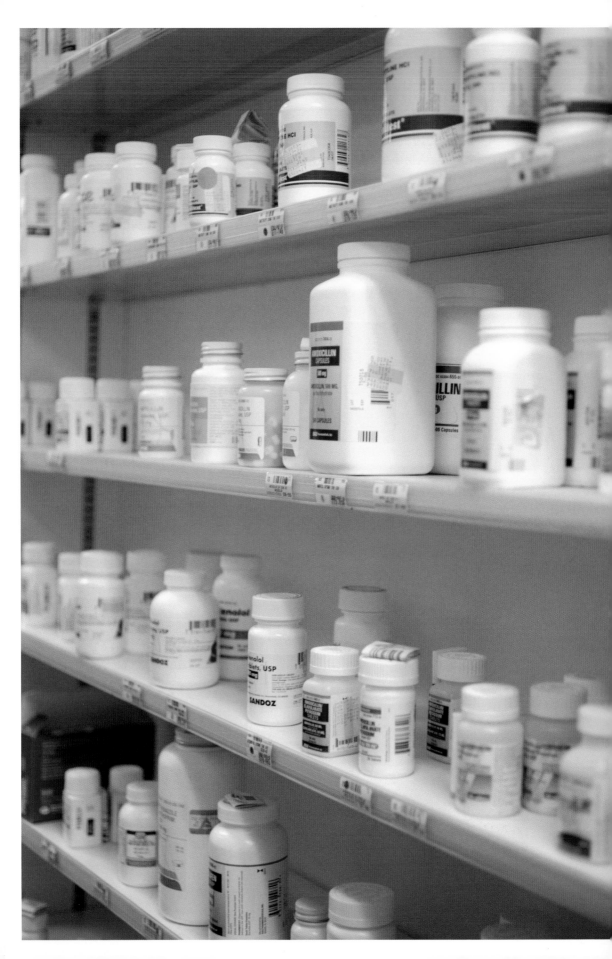

# Chapter 13
# Your Brain and Your Personal Environment

In theory, doctors are scientists and scientists, by and large, believe in the theory of evolution. In fact, scientific organizations hold so strongly to the belief in evolution that they have even excluded and denied jobs to scientists who hold creationist views.[1] One wonders what they would think today of luminaries such as Isaac Newton—the founder of modern physics—or Max Planck—the founder of quantum mechanics. Both men were quite religious. But I digress.

Given that most doctors understand and believe in the theory of evolution, their approach to treating mental health issues is perplexing. Fully 10 percent of all Americans over the age of twelve are currently taking a prescription antidepressant medication.[2] These prescriptions are also accompanied by prescriptions for tranquilizers. According to data from 2010, in that one year alone sixty million prescriptions were issued for tranquilizers.[3] Doctors explain the necessity of these prescriptions by saying they are needed to treat an imbalance of neurotransmitters in the brain.

I don't doubt that there are a lot of anxious or depressed people out there, and this obviously requires attention. But anyone with even a basic understanding of evolution won't buy the idea that tens of millions of Americans are wandering around with an abnormality in their neurotransmitters that requires medication to fix. If cavemen woke up in the morning too depressed to leave the cave or were too anxious to hunt, they starved and their genes

---

[1] P. Sharpe, "Big Bang," *Texas Monthly (Emmis Communications)* 19, no. 1 (1991): 40–43.

[2] "One in 10 Americans Use Antidepressants, Most Don't See a Therapist," *ABC News*, October 19, 2011.

[3] "Drug Abuse Recognition Training," *Talbot*; available at www.drugrecognition.com/Use%20Statistics.htm.

weren't passed on. Does any animal in its natural environment require an antidepressant prescription to avoid suicide?

Clearly, the problem is one of environment rather than evolution. Antidepressants aren't vitamins, and depression isn't caused by Prozak deficiency, nor is anxiety caused by Valium deficiency. There are a lot of environmental factors within our control that definitely affect conditions such as anxiety and depression. For example, both sugar consumption and trans fat consumption as well as the amount of sleep and exercise we get—and how much time we spend watching TV—contribute to the risk of developing these conditions. For many people, gluten and generalized inflammation are contributing factors. The solution is to cure the cause rather than to declare millions of people to have "neurotransmitter imbalances" and pump them full of drugs.

This same situation applies to amphetamines such as Ritalin being prescribed to children. About 19 percent of high school-age boys are diagnosed with ADHD, and about 10 percent of high school-age boys are on these drugs.[4] Again, a caveman hunter who couldn't sit still and pay attention while waiting out his quarry starved. Meanwhile, there are studies linking food additives, insufficient omega-3 intake, excessive television watching, insufficient exercise, and various other easily controlled environmental factors to ADD/ADHD.

Meanwhile, mind-altering drugs prescribed by doctors, including painkillers, tranquilizers, and stimulants, killed 37,485 people in 2009—exceeding the number of deaths by car accidents and even violence and accidents involving firearms. And the vast majority of those deaths were *not* intentional suicides.[5]

To some degree, drugs may be overprescribed or certain conditions may be overdiagnosed. And in the case of stimulants, it's possible that our school system simply has no tolerance for normal

---

[4] U.S. Centers for Disease Control, National Survey of Children's Health 2011–2012.

[5] R. Ricker, "Why Medical Prescriptions May Be Killing Thousands of Americans Every Year," *Huffington Post*, October 8, 2011.

male behavior and has no idea how to channel youthful male exuberance productively.[6, 7, 8, 9]

But at the same time, nobody can deny that the symptoms exhibited by people who are depressed, anxious, or unable to pay attention are quite real and seriously impair their quality of life. Even though it would be easy to blame skyrocketing prescription rates on drug companies or credulous doctors, it would be erroneous to do so. Drug companies obviously have a profit motive, but nobody from the drug company comes to someone's house, holds that person at gunpoint, and forces him or her to make an appointment with the doctor claiming to be depressed. People go to the doctor because they are truly having difficulties that adversely affect their lives.

I am sure that, to some small degree, humans have always had mental illnesses. But we haven't had an *epidemic* of people allegedly needing psychoactive medications until the advent of processed foods and television.

Obviously, our society has changed in various ways with unprecedented rapidity. Just as it can take a hundred years to evaluate the potential harms of introducing a substance such as trans fats to the diet, it can take a long time to see the effects of social changes. And just as evaluation of substances can be inhibited by politics, honest evaluation of the impact of social changes can be inhibited too. We can look all around and see real problems though—whether it be the grass-eaters of Japan and men on marriage strike in America causing reproductive rates to fall year after year. Nearly a quarter of adults between eighteen and thirty-five in

---

[6] D. Flynn, "The Drug War on Boys," *American Spectator*, April 5, 2013.

[7] C. Sommers, *The War Against Boys: How Misguided Feminism Is Harming Our Young Men* (New York: Touchstone, 2000).

[8] P. Tyre, *The Trouble with Boys: A Surprising Report Card on Our Sons, Their Problems at School, and What Parents and Educators Must Do* (New York: Three Rivers Press, 2008).

[9] L. Sax, *Boys Adrift: The Five Factors Driving the Growing Epidemic of Unmotivated Boys and Underachieving Young Men* (New York: Basic Books, 2009).

the United States are living with their parents, and almost a third are out of work as I write this.

In 100 years we went from horses and buggies on dirt roads to traffic jams on eight-lane superhighways. In that same time we went from the telegraph to looking at videos on our cell phones. We went from bolt-action rifles to nuclear umbrellas. We went from correspondence by letters taking weeks to arrive to SMS messaging in which an angst-ridden teenager reads dire import into a friend's failure to answer a text message within mere minutes.

The above just scratches the surface. I'm quite sure the general milieu in which we live, having changed so much, is having an effect on mental health simply because it differs so starkly from the small groups and lifestyle in which we evolved. I can't even begin to address such issues in a book on diet. And, really, I don't believe it is necessary because to a very substantial degree we all control our own environment with our choices.

There are things we can control, and there are things we can't control. But even when it comes to things we can't control, we have the ability to control our own reactions. We can also expand the amount of our lives over which we have control.

## This Is Your Brain on Garbage

A while ago the U.S. Government sponsored a series of anti-drug advertisements featuring a hot frying pan and stating, "This is drugs." Then, an egg was broken into the frying pan, and the announcer said, "This is your brain on drugs." After a short pause, the announcer asked, "Any questions?" Though I'm sure people who were stoned found the advertisement hilarious, the point was nevertheless valid.

The blood-brain barrier is a myth, or at least an inaccurate concept. The general idea of the blood-brain barrier is that the barrier doesn't allow anything harmful to pass, or at least that nothing we eat passes directly. But the permeability of this barrier is easily demonstrated by the effects of hundreds of drugs that act directly upon the brain. If the barrier were so effective, these drugs would not get through.

Yet, in spite of the common-sense evidence that hundreds if not thousands of compounds are able to affect the brain, medical science in general sees the brain and body as separate systems in spite of their profound interdependencies and interactions. As a result, most people do not realize just how substantively our brains are affected by what we eat.

Though eating a high-carbohydrate and/or low fat diet doesn't have an effect on the brain that is quite as dramatic as an overdose of barbiturates, there is considerable evidence that excess carbohydrate consumption (usually in the form of grains) combined with inadequate dietary fat intake is the single largest causative factor of depression. Though the specifics of the mechanism by which this causation takes place are not yet known, the epidemiology of the matter is quite clear.

In fact, the relationship has been widely known, and studies have been published in peer-reviewed publications for more than thirty years. In 1990, for example, two researchers at Texas A&M published a study[10] on using diet to treat depression in which sucrose and caffeine were withheld in one group versus a group in which red meat and artificial sweeteners were withheld. Patients in the first group showed dramatic positive results. Though the confounding variable of caffeine was also present, this study was not alone.

In 1976, Dr. Richard Kunin published a study on using diet to treat anxiety, depression, and dysperception among a group of outpatients, 82 percent of whom experienced an amelioration of symptoms in response to carbohydrate restriction.[11] In 2004, a similar study was done on rats, demonstrating the efficacy of carbohydrate restriction in diminishing depression.[12]

The standard cholesterol-lowering diet prescribed by doctors is very high in carbohydrates and low in fats. Saturated fats from

---

[10] L. Christensen and R. Burrows, "Dietary Treatment of Depression," *Behavior Therapy* 21, no. 2 (1990): 183–93.

[11] R. Kunin, "Ketosis and the Optimal Carbohydrate Diet: A Basic Factor in Orthomolecular Psychiatry," *Orthomolecular Psychiatry* 5, no. 3 (1976): 203–11.

[12] P. Murphy *et al.*, "The Antidepressant Properties of the Ketogenic Diet," *Biological Psychiatry* 56 (2004): 981–83.

animals tend to be replaced by omega-6 polyunsaturated fats from sources such as soybean oil. This diet is accompanied by an increase in rates of depression. In fact, the suicide rates of people on the diet are so high that any decrease in mortality it may incidentally achieve is more than canceled by the increase in suicides.[13,] [14] Though that effect has been somewhat controlled through the rather liberal application of antidepressants in affected populations, at least some researchers have delved to find the underlying cause rather than be satisfied to throw more chemicals at the problem.

Excessive carbohydrates are certainly one of the culprits, but another is the distinct lack of DHA—an animal-made form of omega-3 fatty acid[15]—in the diets of those restricting fat intake, combined with an increase in omega-6 fatty acids. A comprehensive review of the literature stated the matter clearly enough that even a doctor could understand it.

> In major depression, all studies revealed a significant decrease of the polyunsaturated omega-3 fatty acids and/or an increase of the omega-6/omega-3 ratio in plasma and/or in the membranes of the red cells. In addition, two studies found a higher severity of depression when the level of polyunsaturated omega-3 fatty acids or the ratio omega-3/omega-6 was low. Parallel to these modifications, other biochemical perturbations have been reported in major depression, particularly an activation of the inflammatory response system, resulting in an increase of the pro-inflammatory cytokines (interleukins: IL-1b, IL-6 and interferon g) and eicosanoids (among others, prostaglandin E2) in the blood and the CSF of depressed patients.[16]

---

[13] H. Endelberg, "Low Cholesterol and Suicide," *Lancet* 339 (1992): 727–29.

[14] R. E. Morgan *et al.*, "Plasma Cholesterol and Depressive Symptoms in Older Men," *Lancet* 341 (1993): 75–79.

[15] J. R. Hibbeln and N. Salem Jr., "Dietary Polyunsaturated Fatty Acids and Depression: When Cholesterol Does Not Satisfy," *American Journal of Clinical Nutrition* 62, no. 1 (1995): 1–9.

[16] A. Colin *et al.*, "[Lipids, depression and suicide]," *Encephale* 29, no. 11 (2003): 49–58. Review. In French.

In other words, an increase in the amount of omega-6 fatty acids (such as from corn oil, soybean, oil, or other industrial seed oils) and/or insufficient intake of animal-made omega-3 fatty acids (from sources such as seafood) are a major contributor to the poor mental state of people.

But wait! There's more! As discussed in the chapter on grains, gluten causes inflammation in 80 percent of people and generates antibodies in 30 percent of people. Less than 1 percent of people are sufficiently adapted to gluten that it should be considered safe in their diet. Cytokines—the markers of inflammation—are produced in response to the ingestion of gluten, and these most assuredly pass the blood-brain barrier contributing to depression.[17]

And there is yet one more respect in which garbage foods contribute to anxiety and depression: your gut bacteria. Though this fact isn't covered in basic anatomy in elementary school, there is a complex of neurons in your gut that is so extensive many scientists refer to it as "the second brain."[18]

Scientists were surprised to discover that most communication between the gut and brain via the vagus nerve—90 percent of it—goes from the gut to the brain instead of the other way around.

Therefore, the bacteria in your gut and the state of your gut can directly affect your mood. In 2011, researchers confirmed this fact.[19] A recent study of thirty-six women demonstrated that the bacterial content of the gut has wide-ranging effects on our perceptions and feelings.[20]

---

[17] O. J. Schiepers, M. C. Wichers, and M. Maes, "Cytokines and Major Depression," *Progress in Neuropsychopharmacology & Biological Psychiatry* 29, no. 2 (2005): 201–17. Erratum in *Progress in Neuropsychopharmacology & Biological Psychiatry* 29, no. 4 (2005): 637–38.

[18] M. Gershon, *The Second Brain: The Scientific Basis of Gut Instinct and a Groundbreaking New Understanding of Nervous Disorders of the Stomach and Intestines* (New York: Harper, 1998).

[19] "Gut Bacteria Linked to Behavior: That Anxiety May Be in Your Gut, Not Your Head," *Science Daily*, May 17, 2011.

[20] K. Tillisch *et al.*, "Consumption of Fermented Milk Product with Probiotic Modulates Brain Activity," *Gastroenterology* 144, no. 7 (2013): 1394–401.

When you eat junk such as concentrated sugars, grains, and industrial oils, you alter the content of your gut bacteria, and when you do that, you change the sensory stimulus of millions of sensory neurons sending information and updates to the brain.

The bottom line is that the very diet most people would tell you to eat is a major cause of endogenous depression. You do not need grains and sugars such as sucrose in your diet, and you most definitely do not need industrial vegetable oils. Not only is this garbage suicide to eat because of its role in heart disease and cancer but it could also make you so depressed you commit suicide before these diseases fully manifest. They are garbage and nonfood, and are consumed at one's peril.

This, therefore, answers the question about the geometric rise in the rates of depression and anxiety. Just as cancer and heart disease have grown in response to official food recommendations, so have anxiety and depression.

## This Is Your Brain on the Idiot Box

My father has always called TV "the idiot box," and he restricted my TV watching to one hour weekly from childhood all the way through my graduation from high school. It sounds strict, but I am eternally grateful.

As it turns out, watching television is not a healthy activity, and there is a dose-dependent relationship in that the more it is watched, the more harm it does. There are many theories about why it is harmful, spanning all the way from repeated activation of the orienting response, through the sheer sedentary nature of the activity. Despite debate on the theories of the mechanism of harm, no serious researcher disputes that the harm exists.

The increased risks of obesity as it relates to TV are well –known, and I won't rehash them here, but fewer people are aware of the risks TV presents for mental health.

Though there is no link in terms of TV being a *causative* mechanism for anxiety, there is a lot of data demonstrating that TV viewing tends to exacerbate anxiety. Just putting the words "television" and "anxiety" into an Internet search engine turns up examples such as forum posts by anxious people who claim TV makes them more anxious and serious academic studies of the phenomenon. The fact that television has this effect is not a surprise to one commentator who states:

> Many of you have already figured it out; television creates stress—period. Commercial television is designed and intended to create stress for the simple reason that stressed-out people buy things to sedate or distract themselves—or to solve the problems the television tells them they have. This form of mass-hypnosis has been so effective, there are now thousands of television channels; and, a new mass-market has been generated by creating unrealistic self-images and low self-esteem with artificial images of artificial people—and the answer to your problems just a toll-free telephone call away.[21]

The linkage to depression is more profound, with a longitudinal study demonstrating that the more someone watches TV as a teen, the more likely the person is to become depressed as an adult.[22] And when it comes to younger children, the damage from watching TV can create lifelong impediments. Dr. David Perlmutter summarized a lot of research (validated by the American Pediatric Association) in an article stating that TV time for kids can harm their mathematical, social, and language development—sometimes dramatically.[23]

Even when using educational programming, TV viewing retards a baby's development.[24] And as children get older, the more TV they watch, the more it hurts their chances of ever graduating

---

[21] P. Koemer, "Television Is Designed and Intended Tto Create Anxiety, Stress, and Low Self-Esteem," *EzineArticles.com*; available at http://ezinearticles.com.

[22] B. Primack *et al.*, "Association Between Media Use in Adolescence and Depression in Young Adulthood: A Longitudinal Study," *Archives of General Psychiatry* 66, no. 2 (2009): 181–88.

[23] D. Perlmutter, "Brain Development: How Much TV Should Children Watch?" *Huffington Post*, December 5, 2010.

[24] N. Shute, "TV Watching Is Bad for Babies' Brains," *US News*, December 9, 2010.

from college.[25] Part of the reason for this is that watching TV permanently rewires a child's brain, thereby dramatically increasing the risk of developing ADD/ADHD.[26]

Television is clearly something novel in human experience, and its use has well-documented adverse effects that you probably won't hear about on the evening news for obvious reasons. For this reason, it should be dealt with using caveman caution or caveman moderation for adults, should be avoided altogether for infants and toddlers, and should be severely limited for kids and teens.

## This Is Your Brain Without Sleep

Not only does inadequate sleep (defined as less than six hours daily for an adult) increase the risk of obesity, diabetes, and heart disease[27] but it also increases the risk of death from all causes,[28] and adversely affects the brain in numerous ways. For example, a study of young adults determined that insufficient sleep triples the risk of developing psychological distress, including anxiety, depression, and even bipolar disorder.[29]

Adults who chronically get inadequate sleep are four times as likely to develop depression and an astonishing twenty times more likely to develop anxiety or panic disorders.[30]

For the men out there, inadequate sleep makes your body produce more cortisol, and cortisol blocks both the production and

---

[25] A. Gosline, "Watching TV Harms Kids' Academic Success," *New Scientist*, July 4, 2005.

[26] D. Christakis *et al.*, "Early Television Exposure and Subsequent Attentional Problems in Children," *Pediatrics* 113, no. 4 (2004): 708 –13.

[27] "Lack of Sleep Is Linked to Obesity, New Evidence Shows," *Science News Daily*, April 17, 2012.

[28] A. N. Vgontzas *et al.*, "Insomnia with Short Sleep Duration and Mortality: The Penn State Cohort," *Sleep* 33, no. 9 (2010): 1159–64.

[29] N. Glozier *et al.*, "Short Sleep Duration in Prevalent and Persistent Psychological Distress in Young Adults: The DRIVE Study," *Sleep* 33, no. 9 (2010): 1139–45.

[30] D. Neckelmann *et al.*, "Chronic Insomnia as a Risk Factor for Developing Anxiety and Depression," *Sleep* 30, no. 7 (2007): 873–80.

effectiveness of your testosterone, thereby lowering your sex drive, making it hard for you to lose excess weight and lowering your general attractiveness.[31] Testosterone is also linked to the female sex drive, so the excess cortisol from inadequate sleep doesn't do women any favors either.

## This Is Your Brain Without Exercise

The physical benefits of exercise are tremendous, reducing the risk of nearly all serious diseases, but the mental benefits may be even more impressive. Studies show that exercise increases the levels BDNF in the brain, increasing memory and the ability to perform complex tasks.[32]

Though exercise is underutilized as a treatment for depression, it has been shown to be an effective treatment for mild to moderate depression as well as anxiety disorders—along with making people more resilient against such disorders in the first place.[33] Exercise likewise reduces stress, improves self-esteem, and improves sleep.

If you have the ability to exercise outside, you are better off doing so. Although all exercise has benefits, studies show that exercise conducted outside has even greater benefits for mental health compared with exercise done inside.[34, 35]

---

[31] M. Rantala *et al.*, "Evidence for the Stress-Linked Immunocompetence Handicap Hypothesis in Humans," *Nature Communications* 3, article no. 694, February 21, 2012.

[32] É. W. Griffin *et al.*, "Aerobic Exercise Improves Hippocampal Function and Increases BDNF in the Serum of Young Adult Males," *Physiology & Behavior*104, no. 5 (2011): 934–41.

[33] A. Ströhle, "Physical Activity, Exercise, Depression and Anxiety Disorders," *Journal of Neural Transmission* 116, no. 6 (2009): 777–84.

[34] M. G. Berman, J. Jonides, and S. Kaplan, "The Cognitive Benefits of Interacting with Nature," *Psychological Science* 19, no. 12 (2008): 1207–12.

[35] E. M. Simonsick *et al.*, "Just Get Out the Door! Importance of Walking Outside the Home for Maintaining Mobility: Findings from the Women's Health and Aging Study," *Journal of the American Geriatrics Society* 53, no. 2 (2005): 198–203.

## This Is Your Brain Without Sunshine

Most people in North America don't get enough sun and don't eat foods that will provide natural vitamin D in its stead. As a result, the lack of vitamin D increases our risks of everything from obesity and cancer to arthritis.[36]

Everybody needs sunshine for his or her health, and sunshine viewed through a window doesn't cut the mustard, because you need the sun *actually shining on your skin.* In the Northern United States, if you are very light-skinned, you only need twenty to thirty minutes daily on skin normally exposed by clothing.

Getting even that small amount of sun can be difficult in the winter in places like New England where we might not get direct sunlight for days on end. In that event, a vitamin D supplement is one of the very few supplements I recommend.

If you are black, your skin blocks sun much more effectively, and as a result you need a lot more sun in order to get adequate vitamin D—as much as twenty-five times more sun. A bit of math tells you that twenty-five times twenty minutes equals 500 minutes, or more than eight hours a day. Obviously, this isn't even close to practical for most people, and that's why there is an epidemic of vitamin D deficiency among black people in the United States. Especially if you live in the Northern parts of the country, you absolutely need to be taking a vitamin D supplement. Millions upon millions of black people have died prematurely because of lack of awareness of this easily solved problem. For more information about this epidemic and its tragic (and easily prevented) human costs, please see Ms. Allison-Francis's book *Correcting the Vitamin D Deficiency Epidemic: Strategies to Fight Diseases and Prolong Life for Black People.*

But this chapter is about your brain, and given the number of people who get the blues in winter, it isn't surprising to discover that there is a link between vitamin D deficiency and depression.[37] One

---

[36] J. Dowd, *The Vitamin D Cure* (Hoboken, NJ: John Wiley & Sons, 2012)

[37] D. Archer, "Vitamin D Deficiency and Depression," *Psychology Today,* July 11, 2013.

recent study on three severely depressed women showed very positive results from vitamin D supplementation after three months.[38]

Incidentally, vitamin D from the sun is better than vitamin D from supplements because the effect of the sun lasts longer in terms of serum vitamin D concentrations.[39]

## The Caveman Lifestyle and Your Brain

The message of this chapter can be summarized like this: Most of the mental health issues we are treating with psychoactive drugs are either caused or exacerbated by environmental factors in modern life that *we can control.* This includes eating too much carbohydrate (especially in the form of grain and sugar), eating insufficient omega-3, eating too much omega-6 from industrial oils, watching too much TV, getting insufficient sleep, being too sedentary, and not getting enough sun.

Research indicates that correcting these problems will, over time, either cure or prevent the most common psychological ailments for which we take medications, including anxiety, depression, panic disorders, ADD, and ADHD. Patience and persistence are required because it can take anywhere from six to twelve weeks of consistent application to see clear benefits.

---

[38] S. Pathak *et al.*, "Vitamin D Deficiency (VDD) and Major Depressive Disorder (MDD): A Causal or Casual Association?" *Endocrine Reviews* 33, (2012): SAT-377.

[39] M. F. Holick, "Vitamin D and Sunlight: Strategies for Cancer Prevention and Other Health Benefits," *Clinical Journal of the American Society* of *Nephrology* 3, no. 5 (2008): 1548–54.

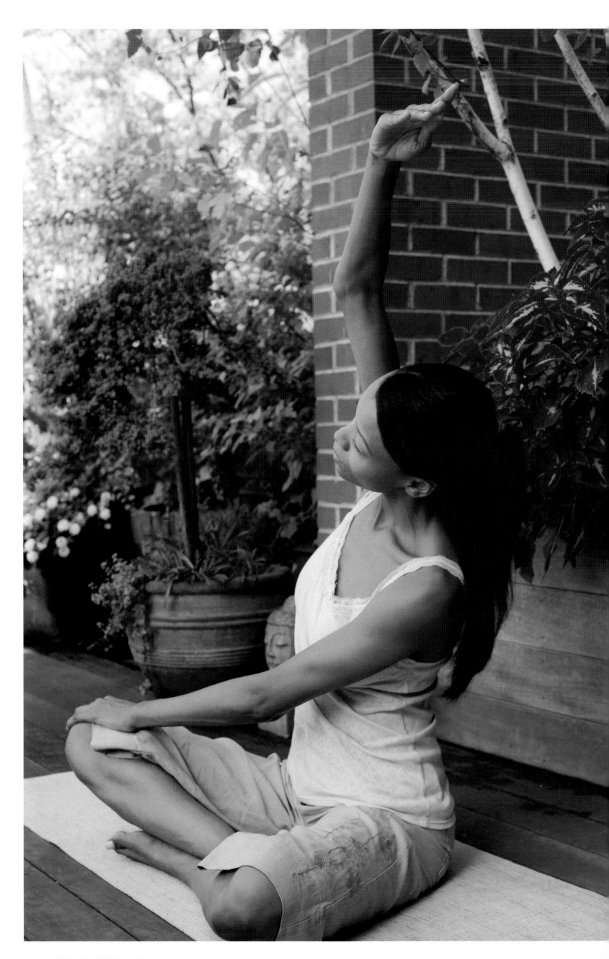

# Chapter 14
## Baseline Caveman Fitness

Anyone who has ever been in a romantic relationship realizes that people are wonderful, horrible, and so incredibly complex as to defy all attempts at understanding.

At every stage in the growth of our understanding, we think we have it all figured out only to find that there is yet more undiscovered. In a simple sense, the genes in our DNA affect many of our personal attributes. Some of our attributes, such as blood type or the color of our eyes, are clearly based in chromosomal DNA and can even be predicted based on the attributes of our parents.

But the deeper we dig, the more we discover that there is more to it than that. Specifically, the science of epigenetics is built upon the discovery that various aspects of our environment (and even our parent's environment and our prenatal hormonal environment) control which of our genes get expressed, how they are expressed, and even how our brain cells are wired. Some epigenetic changes are even as heritable as genes for the next generation. So even though our genes may define a range of expression or the absolute limits of potential, it is within our powers to define just how much of our potential we actually achieve.

This is pretty important. Take two people, one of whom has greater genetic potential in a given arena of performance. Pretend that the person with the greater potential sits in front of soap operas munching potato chips all day while the one with the lesser potential eschews the tube in favor of physical training and eats a decent diet. At the end of a year or five years, which one has the greater absolute performance? The latter, of course.

One thing most people do not realize as they watch elite athletes on television is that all of us with very rare exceptions are born with impressive athletic abilities that we simply have not developed. Our ancestors had to escape from lions, hunt mastodons, and leap into trees at a single bound to avoid becoming a predator's lunch. Maybe you look in the mirror while naked and think it is impossible, but nothing could be further from the truth. You were born to have the body of a gymnast or a sprinter, and you can have that body even if you are old enough to retire.

You might have already dismissed what I am saying because you believe it will take an inordinate amount of time, an expensive gym membership, and a personal trainer along with five years of effort to achieve such a result. That would certainly be true if we approached exercise in the orthodox way, but instead, just as with diet, we will take notes from our ancestors. When approaching exercise as our ancestors did, impressive results can be ours without a gym, with very small expense, and without spending endless hours.

The above applies to people who are healthy overall, even though they may be substantially overweight. But in some cases, it doesn't apply because people have gone so far down the road of morbid obesity, arthritis, or other chronic disease that practically every system in their bodies is stressed. People in such a condition *can* achieve positive results, but it will take longer and requires medical oversight. Look at yourself honestly, and apply common sense. That having been said, the techniques I am about to put forward have been used successfully—and without killing anybody—for cardiac rehabilitation in people who have undergone bypass surgery. So once you have your physician's clearance for strenuous exercise, the only thing standing between you and the body of your dreams is effort.

At first, it is hard to stick to anything that involves effort. But all you have to do is stick with it for a couple of weeks, and after that it becomes a lot easier. The exercise pumps chemicals into your body, such as endorphins, that even make it addictive in a positive sense, and after a couple of weeks you'll start to see positive changes that will further reinforce your continued progress.

If you look at the cover of magazines at the supermarket checkout, there seems to be an appeal to implausible quick fixes: lose two dress sizes in seven days while eating chocolate cake, firm up your flabby arms in five minutes a day, lose that spare tire in just three weeks. While these claims may move magazines off the shelves and into shopping carts, you can look all around you and see that they don't work. What I'm presenting here is not a quick fix, though you may see quick results at first. Rather, I am putting forward a lifetime plan based on solid science as well as our ancestral model.

## Epigenetics of Exercise

Every cell in your body that has a nucleus has the same DNA.[1] Skin cells, however, act quite differently from muscle cells or brain cells. Though they have a great deal in common because they have the same DNA, they behave differently based upon which genes are turned on and which are turned off. If you've watched the science news, you've recently seen stories of scientists taking discarded cells from urine, turning them into undifferentiated stem cells (a stem cell is a sort of "blank slate" that can be acted upon to control what it becomes), and then using those stem cells to grow human teeth.[2]

DNA takes its cues on how to behave—how to express itself—from a variety of other factors in the environment. Though this effect is most dramatic in stem cells, every cell in the body can be induced to change its behavior and function based upon external influences. Exercise is an external influence that can profoundly change the functioning of cells in the body, thereby lowering the risk of most diseases of civilization and increasing quality of life in a variety of ways.

Though most research into exercise concentrates on the readily observable facts of its improvements in weight regulation, triglycerides, blood pressure, and similar items, curious researchers have started to ask *why* exercise makes these changes. The

---

[1] The reason for qualifying this statement is that red blood cells do not have a nucleus.

[2] "Urine Used to Create Teeth—Stem Cell Success," *Medical News Today,* July 30, 2013.

answer is that it changes the way our cells work by changing which genes are expressed and the degree of their expression. One study on skeletal muscle demonstrated dramatic genome-wide changes affecting a dozen genes.[3] A similar study on fat cells demonstrated substantial changes in over *7,000* genes.[4]

If you are looking for the "fountain of youth," you have found it right in your own body. The epigenetic changes from regular strenuous exercise not only make you look better and feel better but also retard the aging process and even reduce the risk of cancer[5] while reducing the risk of cognitive decline and Alzheimer's.[6] Exercise is the most powerful medication available, and if big pharmaceutical companies could patent it and charge a fee, getting access to exercise would be incredibly expensive.

Unfortunately for those holding pharmaceutical stocks, you have access to all the exercise you need with minimal equipment and your own body. Learning through the wisdom of our ancestors, you don't need a gym membership, and you don't need to slave away for hours every day either.

## Caveman Exercise

It is instructive to read the journals of explorers like Tasman, Cook, and Dempier (especially the latter) because they often contain intimate details about the lifestyle and activities of the hunter-gatherer people they encountered. In the introduction I described the people as being almost monolithically well fed and

---

[3] M. D. Nitert *et al.*, "Impact of an Exercise Intervention on DNA Methylation in Skeletal Muscle from First-Degree Relatives of Patients with Type 2 Diabetes," *Diabetes* 61, no. 12 (61): 3322–32.

[4] T. Rönn *et al.*, "A Six Months Exercise Intervention Influences the Genome-Wide DNA Methylation Pattern in Human Adipose Tissue," *PLOS Genetics* 9, no. 6 (2013).

[5] F. Sanchis-Gomar *et al.*, "Physical Exercise as an Epigenetic Modulator: Eustress, the "Positive Stress" as an Effector of Gene Expression," *Journal of Strength and Conditioning Research* 26, no. 12 (2012): 3469–72.

[6] P. Kaliman "Neurophysiological and Epigenetic Effects of Physical Exercise on the Aging Process," *Ageing Research Reviews* 10, no. 4 (2011): 475–86.

well muscled. Though their diet was undoubtedly an important aspect of this, their physical activity played an important role as well.

Our preagricultural ancestors did not live on perfectly flat concrete surfaces, sit at desks all day, and use a car to take them everywhere they went. From a very early age, they had to develop a sense of balance, substantial flexibility, an aerobic capacity that is impressive by today's standards: they literally needed sufficient strength and speed to outrun a tiger, jump up onto a limb, and pull up their body. If they couldn't do that, they died. We are the inheritors of this capacity, and we all have it. It's just a matter of developing it.

Our ancestors didn't have gymnasiums, weight machines, steroids, treadmills, athletic sneakers, or personal trainers. Though there can be benefits from using the devices made possible by modern technology, it is important to realize that our ancestors had everything they needed to develop impressive bodies just by being themselves. This is our legacy as well. You already have everything you absolutely need in your own body. Anything else is a bonus.

In recent years, scientists and investigators have been exploring the activity patterns of hunter-gatherer peoples more closely. They have observed modern hunter-gatherer groups, read the journals of explorers, and even done archaeological reconstruction. Though there are certainly differences between groups based on what is present in the environment, a number of consistent patterns have emerged from research, and the value of these patterns has been confirmed by modern scientific studies.

## Plenty of Rest

Hunter-gatherers don't sleep next to their cell phones or watch reality TV until midnight, then get up again at 5 AM. They go to bed shortly after sunset and rise with the sun. Throughout most of the year, this gives them at least eight hours of sleep.

But they also get lots of rest during the day, albeit in the form of what we would call low-impact aerobics. They walk where they need to go. When they sit, they don't sit in chairs and instead usually sit on the ground. This latter practice, incidentally, helps build flexibility. Both practices help to prevent back problems, which are ubiquitous in the modern world.

Intensity of exercise is alternated. Though there is always a certain baseline level of moderate activity, a day that requires very intense exercise is followed by a day of relative rest. This is important as the most beneficial changes from exercise occur while your body adapts during the period of recovery rather than during the exercise itself.

Overtraining is a serious problem because it can lead to injury, hurt your immune system, and reduce your progress. So make sure that any high-intensity days are followed by low-intensity days, just as our caveman ancestors did.

## Walking Good, Sitting Bad

Depending on the environment and time of year, hunter-gatherers walk anywhere from 6 km to 16 km (between 3.7 mi. and 10 mi.) daily. A four-mile walk takes an hour at a brisk pace, and quite frankly you might not have time for that given today's time-crunched lifestyles. But that amount of walking isn't all done at once by hunter-gatherers—it is done throughout the day. Furthermore, you don't even need the equivalent of 3.7 mi. to gain the benefits. Studies show that just thirty minutes of walking daily—the equivalent of 2 mi.—is enough to lower inflammation and hemostatic markers.[7] So you should establish 3 mi. as your minimum.

You can make sure you get at least three miles of walking daily using a pedometer to measure that you walk at least 6,000 steps and making a couple of simple lifestyle changes. The first is to park far away from stores and other places you are visiting. The extra walking adds up faster than you might believe! Today, I got 600 steps just by parking on the far side of the parking lot of the grocery store. When you consider that people make stops like this

---

[7] *Scandinavian Journal of Medicine and Science in Sports* 18 (2008): 736–41.

every day, just this one simple change can easily cover half of your needed walking.

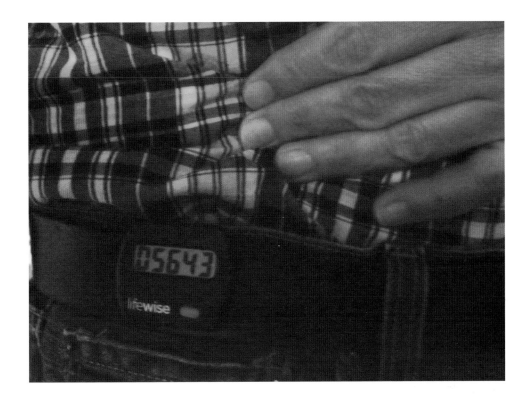

Other changes will depend on your own schedule and work requirements. Taking the long way to the restroom at work, taking a short walk around the building at lunch, and taking the stairs instead of the elevator for a short ride are all possibilities. If, when you get out of work, your pedometer still hasn't clicked on your 6,000th step, just walk around the parking lot at work until it does. Once you get used to how much walking you need to do, you'll develop a feel for it and can ditch the pedometer. Pedometers, incidentally, cost anywhere from $5 to $50, and there are even free pedometer apps available for some smart phones. Just search for free pedometer in the application store for your phone.

Six thousand steps is a baseline. For optimum results, you should shoot for 10,000 steps, or the equivalent of five miles daily. As you know, just about all old-timers claim to have walked five miles to school daily—usually uphill both ways, barefoot on broken glass. That may sound like a lot, and most certainly it would be a large time commitment all at once because it would take about an hour and a half. But if you work it into your day through small changes like parking further away from businesses or taking stairs, you'll find it is quite easily achieved.

Sitting is an independent risk factor for cardiovascular disease, no matter how much you exercise when you are not sitting. It hurts your posture, makes you more prone to weight gain, and increases the risk of developing lower back problems.[8] When I say that sitting is "an independent risk factor," I mean that it increases your risk of having a heart attack (by a whopping 53 percent if you sit all day) whether you smoke or not, whether you eat garbage or not, or whether you exercise or not. The more you stay seated, the more dangerous it becomes.

And here is the thing: all you have to do to negate the damage is to stand up once in a while. It doesn't take much. If you have a job

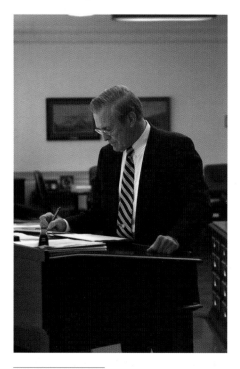

where you are stuck on the phone all day, get a wireless headset and stand up while talking. If you drive long distances to work, stop every hour and just walk around the car a couple of times. As I said, it doesn't take much. Be conscious and make an effort to stand up once in a while—preferably every thirty minutes. I set a small quiet timer at my desk at work.

Just these two simple changes—getting at least 6,000 steps daily and avoiding being seated for long periods—will dramatically reduce your risk of a

---

[8] B. Phillips, "The Most Dangerous Thing You'll Do All Day," *Men's Health*, March 30, 2011.

host of diseases. But it isn't enough to give you optimal physical fitness or to take your body to the next level. To do that, you need to kick things up a notch.

## Proprioception and Balance

Proprioception is defined as "the discrimination of the positions and movements of body parts based on information other than visual, auditory or verbal."[9] It's a big word that describes a person's sense of his or her own body parts and their positions. The standard drunk-driving test of closing your eyes and touching your nose with fingers from both hands tests proprioception.

Proprioception has only been measured in modern times, but studies done on modern populations in the United States consistently show that it declines with age.[10] This has an effect on reaction speeds (thus making activities such as driving more difficult) and contributes to inadvertent injuries due to a lack of postural control. Deficits in proprioception increase the likelihood of practically all accidental injuries. If you don't know where your fingers are without looking, you will more easily cut them in the kitchen. If you don't know where your feet are without looking, you are more likely to trip or fall down stairs. In essence, declining proprioception creates a feedback loop of progressive physical debility.

But many studies indicate that proprioception is adaptive and plastic.[11] In plain language, that means that, in large measure, declines in proprioception can be prevented.

Though many receptors contribute to the aggregate proprioceptive input (including sensors in deep-skin cells and within tendons and ligaments), the primary sensors are integrated with the spindles of skeletal muscle fibers. All of the receptors that

---

[9] Springer Reference, Proprioception

[10] G. Steimach and A. Sirica, "Aging and Proprioception," *Age* 9 (October 1986): 99–103.

[11] D. J. Goble *et al.*, "Proprioceptive Sensibility in the Elderly: Degeneration, Functional Consequences and Plastic-Adaptive Processes," *Neuroscience & Biobehavioral Reviews* 33, no. 3 (2009): 271–78.

contribute to proprioception share in common that they are in locations stimulated by exercise.

Not surprisingly, then, studies have shown that regular exercise dramatically decreases or even eliminates the decline of proprioception with age. A 2003 study of the ability to sense hip position showed no difference in ability between young adults and elderly adults (some as old as eighty-one) who exercise.[12] A study in 2010 demonstrated that elderly adults with a history of exercise have even better proprioception than sedentary young adults.[13]

Though an eighty-one-year-old individual may not be able to compete with a highly trained athlete in the prime of life, the goal of an active and productive life at advanced ages is entirely attainable simply through regular exercise. It is absolutely feasible for the athletic abilities of a person of advanced age to exceed those of an untrained young adult. A great deal of the feebleness seen in the elderly is more a result of inactivity and sedentary lifestyles than age. The exercise need not be overly strenuous; even the slow practice of Tai Chi is sufficient to prevent age-related declines in proprioception.[14]

Related to proprioception is the vestibular system. The core elements of the vestibular system are the semicircular canals in the inner ear that provide our sense of balance. As kids turning somersaults and being bounced on our parents' knees, our vestibular system became highly developed. That system was further honed by playing on monkey bars and swings at the playground. But the vestibular system is a case of "use it or lose it." As adults, people tend to eschew activities that turn them upside down, and the vestibular system loses its development.

---

[12] C. M. Pickard et al., "Is There a Difference in Hip Joint Position Sense Between Young and Older Groups?" Journals of Gerontology Series A: Biological Sciences and Medical Sciences 58, no. 7 (2003): 631–35.

[13] F. Ribeiro and J. Oliveira, "Effect of Physical Exercise and Age on Knee Joint Position Sense," Archives of Gerontology and Geriatrics 51, no. 1 (2010): 64–67.

[14] Xu D, Hong Y, Li J, Chan K (2004). Effect of tai chi exercise on proprioception of ankle and knee joints in old people. Br J Sports Med 38(1):50-54.

Balance has three components: the vestibular system, proprioception, and strength/flexibility. Though deficits in one of the components can often be corrected through strengths in another, the cold reality is that the sedentary lifestyles that cause the loss of vestibular effectiveness also cause a loss of proprioception and strength/flexibility. The good news is that, just as with proprioception, the health of the vestibular system can be enhanced simply through keeping it exercised, and the exercises required are simple.[15]

Because our ancestors didn't have shoes or live on perfectly flat surfaces, they had to exercise their body awareness and balance constantly. We, on the other hand, need a little help. Following is a set of exercises to help you build, maintain, or rebuild your proprioception and vestibular system. These exercises need to be done barefoot for your body to properly work and to achieve maximum benefit.

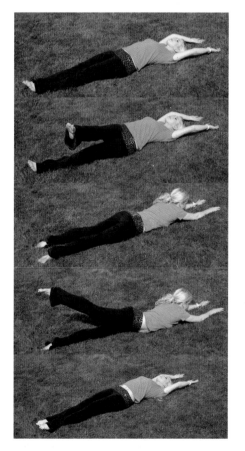

## Exercises to Enhance Your Sense of Balance and Proprioception

### *Rolling Over*

Lie flat on your back with your arms stretched above your head. Raise your right leg, pass it over your left leg, and let your body roll over so you are facedown. While facedown, lift your right leg and pass it over your left leg, then let your body roll over so you are faceup. Repeat this exercise using your left leg.

---

[15] Morley J. Colberg S. *The Science of Staying Young*, McGraw Hill. *2007.*

## Crawling Forward and Backward

Get on your hands and knees, and crawl around as if you were a baby. Make sure to crawl both forward and backward.

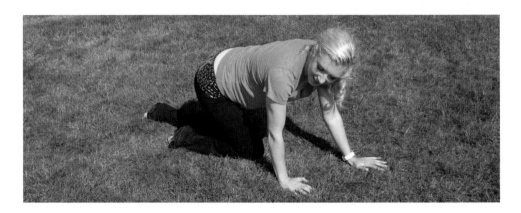

## Standing Tree Pose

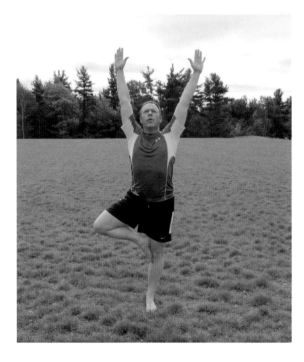

Stand with your feet slightly less than shoulder-width apart and with your hands by your sides. As you raise your right foot to rest against your left knee, bring your hands together in the center of your body and slowly raise them over your head until they separate and you reach for the sky. Stay balanced on one foot for several seconds, then return to your ready pose and repeat with the other leg.

## *Flying Stretch*

Stand with your feet slightly less than shoulder-width apart with your hands by your sides. Raise your right knee to waist level as you raise your hands toward your shoulders. Bend at the waist as you stretch your hands out in front of you and bring your right leg outstretched behind you. In the final position, you look like Superman flying, but supported by your left leg. Hold for up to thirty seconds before slowly returning to the starting position and repeating with the other leg.

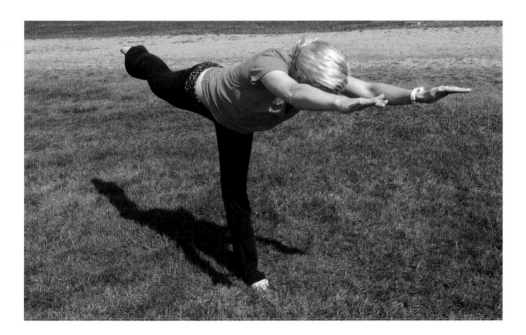

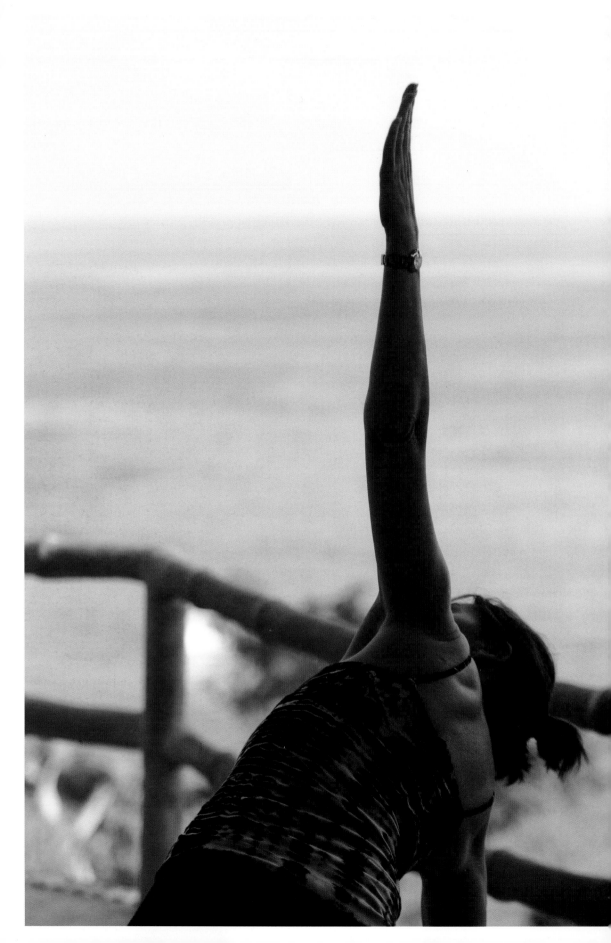

# Chapter 15
# Caveman Flexibility

As mentioned in the previous chapter, your physical ability relies on a combination of proprioception, the vestibular system, and strength/flexibility. If any of these fails, we become frailer, more prone to injury, more tentative in our movements, and less able to live life to the fullest.

The flexibility of cavemen was constantly challenged throughout life, whereas modern lifestyles can protect us from the slightest challenges. This leads to a gradual decline in flexibility and increased risk of injury from even the most undemanding of tasks. Because hunter-gatherers don't sit in cubicles all day then become melded to their couches all night, they maintain flexibility throughout their lives into old age. We can do the same in the modern world through some very modest lifestyle changes.

Flexibility refers to the range of motion around joints. The amount of flexibility available in a given joint is determined by tendons, ligaments, muscles, and bone structure. Each person has individual limits to flexibility that will be different than the limits of other people, though most people other than elite athletes have plenty of room for improvement.

When joints are mentioned, most people think of obvious joints such as those at the knees and elbows, but shoulders, hips, ankles, wrists, neck, feet, hands, and spine also have joints. One of the reasons why sitting for long periods can predispose back injury is because it restricts movement of the dozens of joints in the backbone, thereby causing some of the tendons and ligaments to become unnaturally shortened. Wearing shoes constantly is like putting a cast on your foot, causing the muscles and ligaments to atrophy and making injuries more likely.

Though experts debate the relative merits of various stretching techniques in a fashion reminiscent of debating how many angels can dance on the head of a pin, the evidence indicates that the time-tested approaches work, as do many of the more modern techniques. In essence, so long as used within a margin of safety and preceded by a basic warm-up, any stretching regimen will be beneficial.

The basic warm-up before stretching *should not be skipped* and can be anything from a one-minute walk on a treadmill or up and down the stairs of your house to doing twenty jumping jacks or throwing a series of light punches at a punching bag while doing some footwork. This increases blood flow to the muscles and ligaments, raises their temperature, and primes them for movement so that stretching will be more effective and injury free.

Stretching has to be practiced—ideally daily—to be effective. There are sensors in the muscles and tendons that trigger a reflex that inhibits stretching as a protective mechanism. As you continue to practice stretching, those sensors will reset to encompass new limits, and you'll gain flexibility and range of motion. Don't force any stretches beyond a distinct feeling of stretching. Just take your time, and before you know it, you'll see noticeable results.

Stretching falls into three categories: static, dynamic and ballistic. Though all three approaches to stretching will work to increase flexibility, each works better in some applications than in others.

Static stretches involve using bodyweight or position to hold a joint in place while stretching the muscles at the limit of the their range of motion. The limit of the range should be approached slowly and extended gently without any bobbing or bouncing. The stretch is then held for thirty seconds before the position is relaxed. An example of a static stretch is bending over to touch your toes. The static stretches I'm covering here may look familiar because they can be found in military basic training, warm-ups for track and field, physical education classes, martial arts stretching, and yoga. The back and abdominal stretches using a Swiss ball were contributed by Rob Freeman.

Static stretches are best done following a warm-up, after a workout, or in the evening before bed. Though my track coaches from high school and college would have been shocked at what modern research has revealed, static stretches *do not decrease risk of injury* during athletic endeavors that immediately follow them. (They don't increase the risk of injury either, so my coaches were doing no harm in that respect.) A randomized trial of Army recruits showed no meaningful benefit in terms of injury reduction.[1] A meta-analysis in the *Journal of Athletic Training* echoed that conclusion.[2]

Furthermore, static stretching done immediately before exercise, though it doesn't increase injury risk, can have a substantial negative effect on performance that lasts as long as an hour after the stretches were performed.[3] Static stretches result in a loss of both strength and speed for up to an hour after they have been performed.[4] Therefore, as I have already mentioned, the time and place for static stretches is after a warm-up, after a workout, or before bed. Applied in this way, static stretches will increase flexibility without compromising workouts.

The type of stretching that works best before a workout is *dynamic stretching.* Dynamic stretching uses muscular power and momentum rather than body position, external force, or body weight to elongate muscles and ligaments. The movements of a dynamic stretch are often slow-paced but exaggerated versions of the movements that will be used in a caveman workout.

The range of the dynamic stretch is limited by what the muscles can achieve under control without resorting to bouncing. The range achieved through dynamic stretching is not as great as that attained through static stretches, because it is limited to the range

---

[1] R. P. Pope *et al.*, "A Randomized Trial of Preexercise Stretching for Prevention of Lower-Limb Injury," *Medicine and Science in Sports and Exercise* 32, no. 2 (2000): 271–77.

[2] J. Andersen, "Stretching Before and After Exercise: Effect on Muscle Soreness and Injury Risk," *Journal of Athletic Training* 40, no. 3 (2005): 218–20.

[3] J. Fowles *et al.*, "Reduced Strength After Passive Stretch of the Human Plantar Flexors," *Journal of Applied Physiology* 89, no. 3 (2000): 1179–88.

[4] A. G. Nelson *et al.*, "Acute Effects of Passive Muscle Stretching on Sprint Performance," *Journal of Sports Sciences* 23, no. 5 (2005): 449–54.

that the muscles can fully control. But this is also the factor that makes it a better choice for use prior to a workout.

Because dynamic stretches utilize movement as part of the stretch, they can serve the purpose of both warm-up and stretching protocol at the same time. Unlike static stretches, dynamic stretches reduce the risk of injury[5] without compromising strength or speed.[6]

If you think about it, it's quite likely that our caveman ancestors did the equivalent of dynamic stretching before vigorous exertion and static stretching after the fact. The quiet walk to the hunting area across fallen trees required a dynamic stretch, and sitting on the ground by the campfire recounting hunting stories would have provided a static stretch.

The final type of stretching is ballistic stretching. Ballistic stretching is similar to dynamic stretching in that it uses muscular power, except that it uses momentum and inertia to elongate muscles and ligaments to a degree beyond what can be achieved under completely controlled muscle movement. Though ballistic stretching has been shown to be effective at increasing range of motion and flexibility, it is also likely to create injuries—especially to tissues that have been injured previously.[7]

Ballistic movements of this sort are far better employed when incorporated within plyometric strength exercises. With such exercises, there is enough warm-up to reduce the risk of injury.

---

[5] E. Witvrouw *et al.*, "Muscle Flexibility as a Risk Factor For Developing Muscle Injuries in Male Professional Soccer Players. A Prospective Study," *American Journal of Sports Medicine* 31, no. 1 (2003): 41–46.

[6] T. Yamaguchi and K. Ishii, "Effects of Static Stretching for 30 Seconds and Dynamic Stretching on Leg Extension Power," *Journal of Strength and Conditioning Research* 19, no. 3 (2005): 677–83.

[7] E. Witvrouw *et al.*, "Muscle Flexibility as a Risk Factor for Developing Muscle Injuries in Male Professional Soccer Players. A Prospective Study," *American Journal of Sports Medicine* 31, no. 1 (2003): 41–46.

## Simple Changes

Some simple lifestyle changes can enhance your flexibility. Go barefoot for a little while every day when and where it is safe to do so. This will enhance the flexibility and strength of your feet and ankles while providing valuable proprioceptive feedback.

Sit on the floor instead of in chairs. Sitting on the floor and shifting your weight around as needed will provide a natural stretch for hip flexors, ankles, and other joints.

Stand up periodically from tasks that require being seated in a chair. By standing up periodically you give the tiny tendons, ligaments, and muscles that run between the vertebrae in your back an opportunity to adjust themselves into a more natural state.

## Static Stretching Routine

The following routine is oriented to specifically address the flexibility issues engendered by civilization, such as excessive time sitting in cars and cubicles. It will also extend flexibility suitable for most athletic pursuits as well as an active life. The entire routine should be performed barefoot. Each stretch should be held for thirty to sixty seconds and then gently released. Going through the series once is sufficient, and it will take between ten and fifteen minutes depending on how long you hold the stretches.

Ideally, this routine will be performed after a workout or before going to bed. Alternately, do the routine after a short warm up such as walking up and down a flight of stairs twice or doing twenty jumping jacks. Three times a week is enough, though there is no harm in doing it every day. If you add the standing tree pose and flying stretch from the previous chapter to this routine, it will cover your needs for proprioception and balance exercise as well. If you choose to add those two exercises, add them at the end of the routine.

### *Lying Tree Pose*

Lie flat on your back with your arms stretched out straight above your head. Slowly bring your right foot up so that your right ankle rests slightly above your left knee. Allow your right leg to relax and hang for thirty seconds, then bring your right foot back to the starting position and repeat with the left foot.

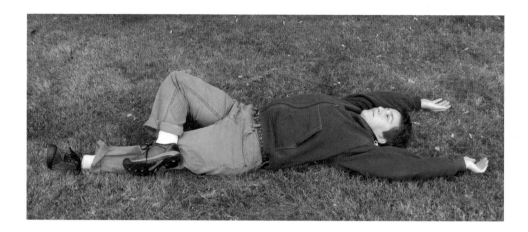

## *Bound Angle Posture*

Lying flat on your back, bring the soles of your feet together and draw them upwards toward your crotch while leaving the edges of your feet in touch with the ground. Allow your legs to relax in this position, and allow gravity to pull your knees toward the floor for thirty seconds before returning to the starting position.

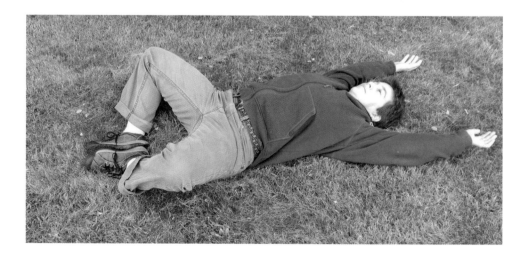

## Prone Hamstring Stretch

Lie flat on your back and bend your knees while drawing your feet toward your butt so that you are in a comfortable knees-raised position. Extend your right leg, and grab your right knee with both hands, gently bringing the knee toward your head until you feel a stretch. Hold it there for thirty seconds, then return to the knees-raised position and repeat with the other leg.

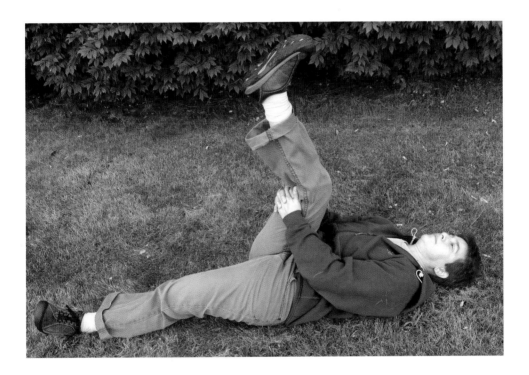

## Prone Gluteus Stretch

Lie flat on your back, and bend your knees while drawing your feet toward your butt so that you are in a comfortable knees-raised position. Bring your right ankle up to rest just below your left knee, then grab your left knee with both hands and gently pull it toward your head until you feel a stretch. Hold it there for thirty seconds, then return to the knees-raised position and repeat with the other leg.

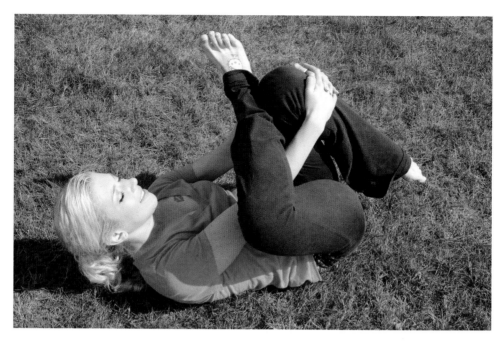

## *Bridging*

From a comfortable knees-raised position, raise your hips so that your knees, hips, and shoulders form a straight line. Hold this position for thirty seconds before relaxing back into a knees-raised position. Repeat once.

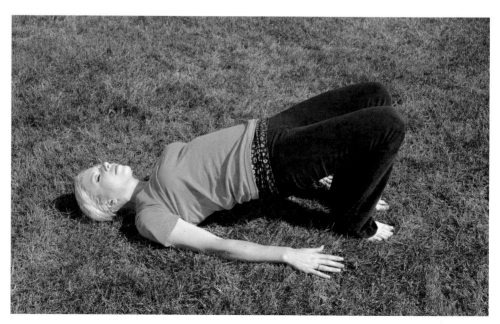

## Cobra

Roll over so that you are lying facedown on the floor. Rest your forearms on the floor even with your shoulders, then press upwards while keeping your waist on the floor so your back will bend. Raise your body up only until you feel a stretch in your abdomen and/or back. As you gain flexibility, use your hands instead of your forearms. Hold for thirty seconds before returning to the starting position.

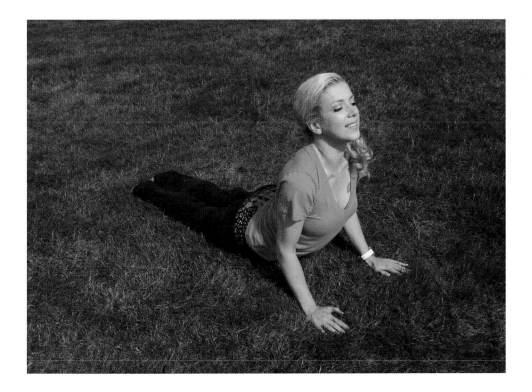

## Back Extension

Get on your hands and knees. Straighten out your right hand and left leg so they are pointing straight away from you, and make small circles in the air with both at the same time for thirty seconds. Then return to your hands and knees, and repeat using your left hand and right leg. If you are having back problems, bend your knee instead of keeping it straight, as this will concentrate the stretch in the muscles most likely contributing to the problem.

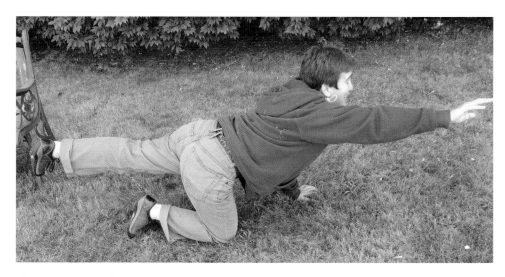

## *Cat Stretch*

While on your hands and knees, arch your back as far as you can comfortably and hold for thirty seconds, then let your back and stomach sag as far as you can and comfortably hold for thirty seconds. You can do another version of the stretch while standing. Bend over and put your palms on the top of your knees, then press your lower back outward and hold for thirty seconds. I find this variant especially useful when taking a break from seated tasks.

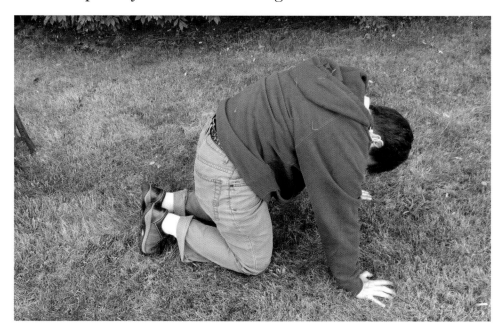

### Buddha Sleeping on Mountain

This stretch uses a Swiss ball. The ball should be at least twenty-one inches in diameter to achieve the proper stretch. Lie across the ball facedown, positioning your abdomen across the ball for greatest stretch and relax your feet and arms so they hang loosely. Because this stretch can compress your diaphragm and ribcage, at first you may feel like you can't breathe. But if you relax and concentrate on forcing your belly outward as you draw in a breath, you'll find you can breathe fine and that breathing enhances the stretch.

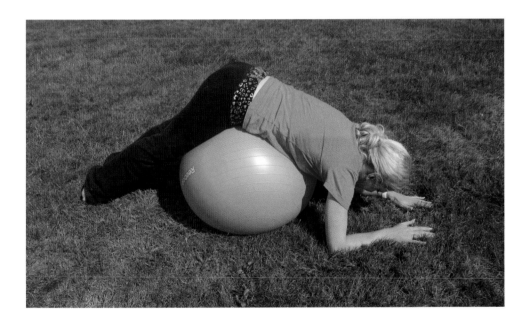

### Bear Awakens in Spring

This stretch uses a Swiss ball. The ball should be at least twenty-one inches in diameter to achieve the proper stretch, and it should be properly inflated. Lie faceup on the ball with your feet on the floor and the ball centered in your lower back. Stretch your hands out above your head and relax so that your hands are moved toward the floor.

Getting into position can be a bit tricky at first, so try this: Sit on the ball with your feet flat on the floor about a foot away from the ball and a bit more than shoulder-width apart. Bring your arms up in front of you so that they are above your head, and arch your back as you let the ball roll from your butt to your lower back and thrust out your hips like you are making a music video. (You may end up on tiptoes if you are short.) Then relax and let your head and arms be pulled toward the floor by gravity. You may have to spread your feet wider to maintain balance.

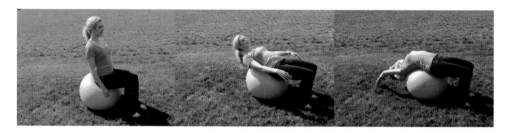

### Forward Bend

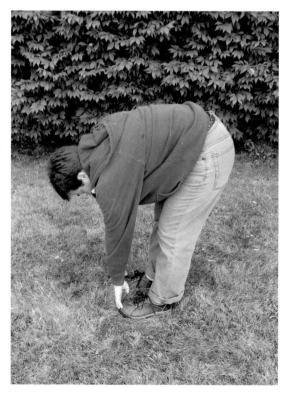

Stand tall with your feet a couple of inches apart. Bend at the waist as your hands reach for your toes or the floor slightly in front of your toes while keeping your knees straight. Reach as far as you can while attaining a comfortable stretch and hold for thirty seconds before returning to the starting position.

### Arm Across

Stand with your feet shoulder-width apart, and

hold both hands straight out in front of you as though you've just pushed something. Using your left hand, grab your right arm just above the elbow, and pull your right arm across your chest. Hold for thirty seconds, then return to the starting position and repeat with the other arm.

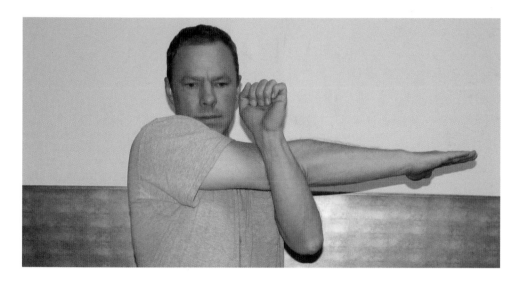

## Flex and Extend Wrists

Stand with your feet shoulder-width apart, and interlace the fingers of your hands with your palms facing away from you. Slowly push your interlaced hands away from you until you feel a gentle stretch. Hold for thirty seconds, and then return to the starting position.

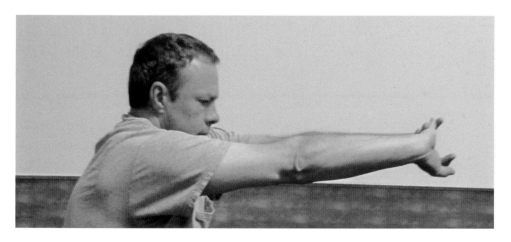

## Reach Back and Turn

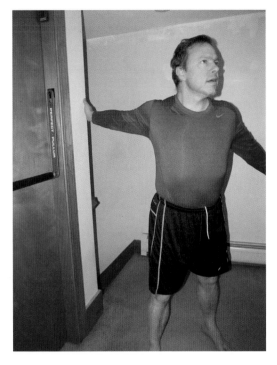

This stretch requires a vertical object that you can grab. A doorjamb, a tree, or any other stable object that is at least as tall as your shoulder will work. Position yourself with your chest even with the object, then extend your right arm at shoulder level and gently hold the object with your right hand. Step forward very slightly until you feel a gentle stretch across your chest. Hold for thirty seconds, and then switch sides.

## Elbow Push

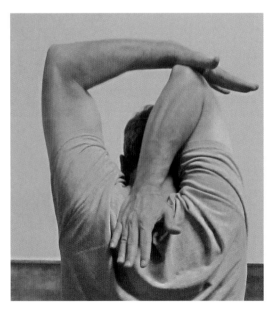

Stand with your feet in a natural position and extend your right arm over your head. Keeping your upper arm pointing upward, bend at the elbow so that your hand touches the middle of your upper back. Then use your left hand to apply gentle downward pressure on your right elbow. Hold for thirty seconds, then repeat with the other arm.

## Head Tilt

People holding their heads in an unnatural position to stare at computer monitors all day damage their necks and head positioning, making them more prone to injury. Stretches for the neck are important to fix

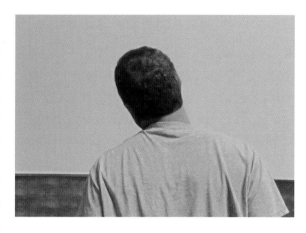

this, but they need to be done very slowly and very gently.

Stand tall with your arms relaxed and hanging at your sides and your head in a straight line with the rest of your body. Use a mirror to check your position if you aren't sure. Slowly tilt your head to the left by bringing your left ear toward your left shoulder until you feel a slight stretch. Hold the position for thirty seconds, return to the starting position, and repeat by tilting your head to the right.

## Head Turn

Stand tall with your arms relaxed and hanging at your sides and your head in a straight line with the rest of your body. Use a mirror to check your position if you aren't sure. Slowly turn your head to the left while

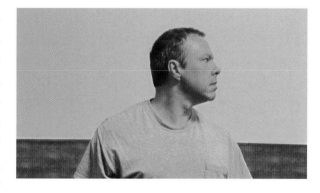

keeping your chin level until you feel a slight stretch. Hold the position for thirty seconds, return to the starting position, and repeat by turning your head to the right.

## Dynamic Stretching Routine

Like the static stretching routine, this routine is oriented toward correcting and preventing the maladies created by civilization. Beyond that, dynamic stretching routines tend to be customized toward the movements of specific sports. Rather than create a limitation, I have created a routine suitable for a combination of kung fu and gymnastics, which are the endeavors requiring the most versatile flexibility. Since I am a kung fu instructor, it's also the arena in which I am most comfortable.

Take it easy with this routine at first, especially if you are unused to exercise. If you have been sedentary for several years, this routine alone may be sufficient as an introductory workout for a couple of weeks. If you are in better condition, it will also serve as a warm-up. The entire routine will take about ten minutes and is best done barefoot if you have a suitable surface.

### *Roll and Reach*

Sit on the floor with your knees bent. Use your hands to grab your knees and bring your thighs close to your chest. Tuck in your chin and roll backward until your shoulder blades touch the floor. Roll back forward, and as you do, extend your legs and bend at the waist while attempting to bring your chest as close to your thighs as you can. Return to the starting position, and repeat for a total of ten repetitions. Perform this exercise carefully and under control so you don't accidentally crack your head on the floor.

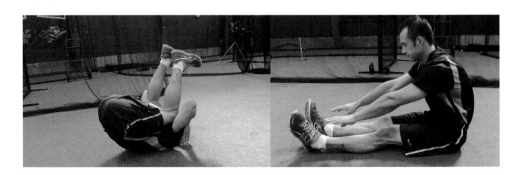

## Table

Sit on the floor with your knees bent and your heels about a palm's width away from touching your butt. Lean back a bit and put your upper body's weight on your hands, which should be resting palm down on the floor about a foot behind you. Gently arch your

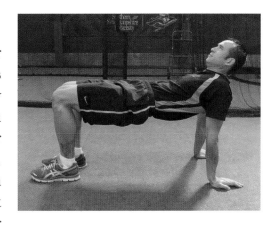

back, and flex your hips outward so that you end up in a table position. Return to the starting position, and repeat for a total of ten repetitions.

Many people find this stretch difficult or even impossible on the first attempt, but don't be discouraged. Every person's body is a bit different, and the exact placement of feet and hands will vary a bit with individual body mechanics. Just get as much range of motion as you can out of the exercise, and each time your body position will become more refined until you can finally do it with ease.

## Push-up Crawl to Standing Position

Start off in a high push-up position. Walk your hands back a little at a time until your are finally in a standing position, bent over with your hands on the floor. Now, walk your hands back out into the high push-up position again. Repeat for a total of five times.

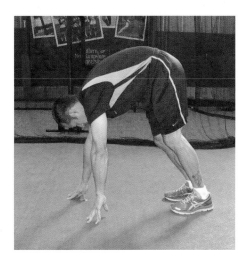

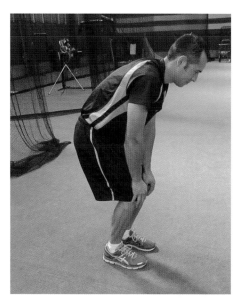

### Knee Circles

Stand with your feet together, then bend at the knees and hips in order to rest your palms on top of your knees. First make a series of clockwise circles with your knees, followed by a series of counterclockwise circles.

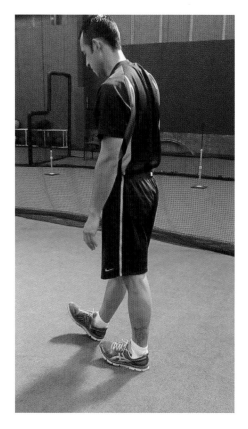

### Heel Walk

Stand with your feet a bit less than shoulder-width apart, then bend your ankles, bringing your toes and the soles of your feet off the ground so that only your heels are touching the ground. Now walk fifteen steps on your heels, then turn around and walk back on your heels. If you are in an area with a space constraint, you can do this stretch walking in place, but it is more beneficial for your calves if you can at least take a couple of steps in each direction.

### Knee to Chest Walk

This is an exaggerated walking motion. With each step, first bring your knee up as close to your chest as you can, then take the stride. Take ten steps in one direction, then turn around and take ten steps back to where you started.

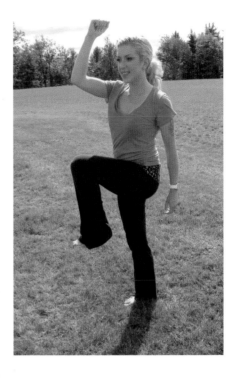

### Carioca

The carioca is a great exercise for building agility and flexibility in your hips and waist. Start off slowly until you get used to the motion, then do it more quickly. Start with your feet shoulder-width apart. Step behind your left leg with your right foot, then take a step to your left with your left foot. Step in front of your left leg with your right foot, and take a step to your left with your left foot. Keep alternating with your right foot first going behind and then in front of your left foot until you've taking ten steps. Then reverse the process as you take steps to the right back to your starting position.

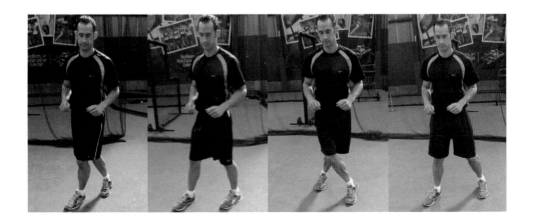

### Straight-Leg Pendulum

Stand with your feet together, then lean slightly to the left and bend your right ankle upward so that your right foot isn't touching the ground. Keeping your right leg straight, swing it back and forth as though it were a pendulum. If you have to hold onto something to keep your balance, that's fine. Do ten swings with your right leg, then reverse the process and do ten swings with your left leg.

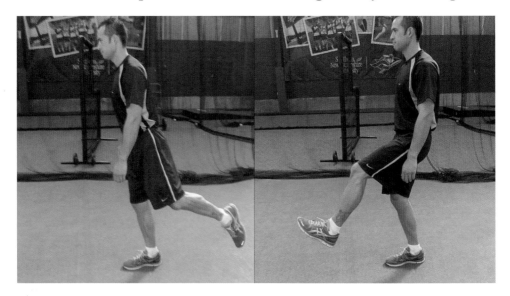

### Cross Reach

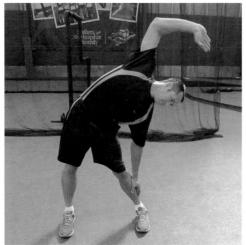

Stand with your feet shoulder-width apart. Cross your right foot across your left, and rest the ball of your right foot on the ground. Reach toward your right knee with your right hand while reaching for the sky with your left hand. Reverse the technique. Repeat five times for each side.

## Chest Expansion

Stand with your feet shoulder-width apart and your hands hanging comfortably at your sides. Raise your arms, put your hands behind your head, just lightly touching your head without pressure, and move your elbows back as far as they can comfortably go. Bring your hands back to the starting position, and repeat five times.

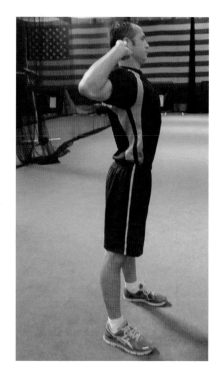

## Windmills

Stand with your feet about 50 percent wider than your shoulders and with your hands above your head. Bend at the waist to touch your left toe with your right hand, return to the starting position, then bend at the waist to touch your right toe with your left hand and return to the starting position again. Repeat five times for each side. Stretch your free arm out behind you as you execute these.

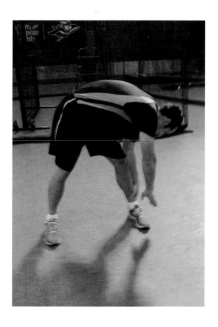

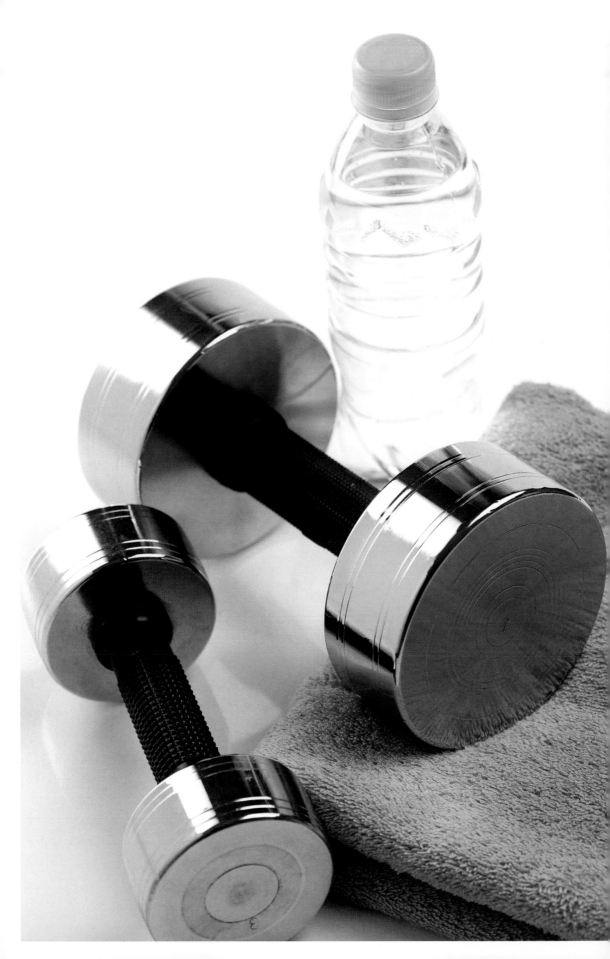

# Chapter 16
# Caveman Strength and Power

In chapters 14 and 15, we covered the necessary background levels of activity and flexibility that are necessary for health and in harmony with our evolution. The topics that remain to be explored are strength, power, aerobic capacity, and cross-training.

Cavemen did not have gyms, weight machines, or carefully calibrated barbells. They hunted prey, ran to avoid becoming prey, climbed over rocks and up trees, carried firewood and food back to camp, and made tools. They also fought with each other. They didn't spend hours in the gym, wear specialized shoes, or run for miles on asphalt. Yet, they had solid functional fitness that in terms of shear athletic ability would put the typical gym denizen to shame.[1]

If you have access to a gym, there are a couple of pieces of gear that may be helpful if used properly. For some people, home life is so chaotic or demanding that they'll never get their fitness routines accomplished unless they set aside time to do them someplace else. So a gym can be handy for that. Also, there can be a certain mindset of mental preparation that is associated with going to the gym that makes it worthwhile. So, while a gym is not necessary, you can go to a gym or health club for your workouts if it suits you.

On the other hand, people are very time-crunched in the modern world. Long work days, traffic, errands, and running around with the kids leave us pressed for time. Many of us can't carve the time out of our schedules for going to the gym, so fitness is best accomplished at home.

So in this chapter, I am approaching fitness the modern caveman way. Though you'll need a couple of inexpensive items that simulate elements of the natural world to make best use of this

---

[1] J. O'Keefe *et al.*, "Organic Fitness: Physical Activity Consistent with Our Hunter-Gatherer Heritage," *The Physician and Sports Medicine* 38, no. 4 (2010): 1–8.

program, most of what you need is included in your own body, and you can build impressive athleticism in about fifteen minutes every other day right in your own home.

Yes, you read that last sentence correctly. Get 6,000–10,000 steps daily in your normal routine, and stand up at your desk once in a while. Then, every other day—so three or four days a week—do ten minutes of dynamic stretching, a fifteen-minute workout, and ten minutes of static stretching (including balance and proprioception exercise), and you are looking at a complete fitness plan that will not only give you an impressive body but also a level of functional strength that will let you get the most out of life all the way into advanced age. At most, you will need thirty-five minutes every other day. Since the average American spends five hours daily glued to the tube, I'm convinced that you can find the time.

## High-Intensity Interval Training Explained

There are many variations of high-intensity interval training (aka HIIT). It seems to have taken thousands of years for us to rediscover, because in fact it is the closest match for how our ancestors achieved their impressive levels of fitness.[2] Just as the discussions of diet earlier in the book demonstrated that the more closely our diet matches the diet of our evolution, the more healthy it is, there is now a mountain of evidence showing that exercise that matches our evolution is the most effective and healthy.

Imagine for a moment that one of your primal ancestors is stalking through the forest in search of a wild pig for dinner. He spies the pig and hurls his spear. The spear finds its target, but the pig takes off running at full speed. Your ancestor takes off after it because it will be easily lost in the underbrush, and he needs to deliver the killing blow so he can eat. He catches up to the pig, which is slowing due to blood loss, pulls the spear out, and delivers a second blow that fells the pig. He picks up the pig, which weighs perhaps eighty pounds, and starts carrying it back to his fellow hunters.

---

[2] Ibid.

On his way back, a tiger notices and gives chase. He drops the pig and takes off for dear life, running at full speed until he can jump to reach the limb of a tree eight feet off the ground. Then he pulls himself up into the tree, climbs up a few more branches for added safety, and waits for the tiger to leave. If he has a sense of humor and has to relieve himself, maybe he pees on the tiger.

At no point during this process did he stop to take his pulse, calculate 80 percent of his maximum heart rate for his age, and slack off or pace himself. He was either at relative rest or going all out and exerting his maximum effort because anything less than maximum effort would have resulted in failure or death.

This is what HIIT is all about. You exert maximum effort for a short amount of time, rest for a short time, and then do it again. Though, as I mentioned, there are many specific approaches to this, such as tabatas, fartleks, whistle drills, and many more, the key concept of maximum effort for a short time followed by a short rest remains the same.

## Is Maximum Effort Safe?

At first blush, going all-out seems like a great way to hurt yourself, but in practice it is self-limiting, so it turns out to be quite safe.

If you are in horrendous condition, just walking up the stairs to your bedroom might constitute maximum heart rate exercise, whereas if you are in better condition you might need to do twenty burpees to achieve maximum heart rate. (Burpees will be described later.) So maximum effort is an adaptive concept that matches you.

According to an article in the *New England Journal of Medicine*, the odds of death from an instance of vigorous exercise are extremely low (less than one in a million), and the more often you engage in vigorous exercise, the lower the risk.[3]

---

[3] C. M. Albert *et al.*, "Triggering of Sudden Death from Cardiac Causes by Vigorous Exertion," *New England Journal of Medicine* 343, no. 19 (2000): 1355–61.

If you have been a couch potato, your odds of sudden cardiac death from vigorous exercise would be higher. Because of this, I want you to do two things. First, have a physical exam, and get your doctor's clearance that there's nothing wrong with your heart. Second, start this program at somewhat less than maximum effort, and work up to it.

A review of the use of high intensity interval training as rehabilitation for patients with heart failure and coronary artery disease concluded that

> HIIT appears safe and better tolerated by patients than moderate-intensity continuous exercise (MICE). HIIT gives rise to many short- and long-term central and peripheral adaptations in these populations. In stable and selected patients, it induces substantial clinical improvements, superior to those achieved by MICE, including beneficial effects on several important prognostic factors (peak oxygen uptake, ventricular function, endothelial function), as well as improving quality of life. HIIT appears to be a safe and effective alternative for the rehabilitation of patients with CAD and HF.[4]

So even though high-intensity interval training is safe enough that it is even used for cardiac rehabilitation of people with heart failure, I recommend that you work up to it—just to be on the safe side.

## Is HIIT Really Better?

If you have been an athlete used to long and grueling workouts, the idea of a fifteen-minute workout being sufficient sounds too good to be true. It is, and it isn't.

When you train for an athletic endeavor, you are training for a very specific task. Though you may incidentally develop whole-body fitness, there are many specifics to a given endeavor that

---

[4] T. Guiraud *et al.*, "High-Intensity Interval Training in Cardiac Rehabilitation," *Sports Medicine* 42, no. 7 (2012): 587–605.

require perfecting. When I ran hurdles in high school and college, we worked a lot on form coming out of the blocks and going over the hurdles, as well as timing for three-stepping the hurdles. You need to practice such skills continuously so they are embedded in muscle memory and are executed by your body without need for conscious thought.

The same applies to martial arts. Workouts for martial arts will take much longer than fifteen minutes because you are executing the same techniques repeatedly so they can be done without need for conscious thought.

There are also specific sports that require very specific physical changes to optimize performance for that sport. That's why you won't see winners of marathons also winning power lifting medals or vice versa.

What this HIIT program using whole-body movement gives you is solid general and functional fitness. It's the kind of fitness you need to run up the stairs when you hear a thump and a baby starts crying, or you are carrying in wood from the woodshed or splitting kindling. It's the fitness of a gymnast or a martial artist rather than the fitness of a bodybuilder or marathoner. (Though in order to *be* a gymnast or martial artist, you'd also have to practice those specific skills. But HIIT will make sure your fitness isn't holding you back.)

But those caveats aside, yes, absolutely—fifteen minutes of HIIT every other day can and will give you phenomenal results. As noted by the researchers cited in the previous section, when compared to MICE (which means plodding on treadmills or elliptical machines at a steady pace for a long time), HIIT improves the function of your heart and blood vessels while increasing your oxygen uptake. But there are even more benefits.

A study in Norway discovered that a single bout of HIIT weekly reduced heart attack risk more than expending 1,000 calories in a so-called aerobic exercise.[5] In a Canadian study, a HIIT program

---

[5] U. Wisløff *et al.*, "A Single Weekly Bout of Exercise May Reduce Cardiovascular Mortality: How Little Pain for Cardiac Gain? 'The HUNT Study, Norway,'" *European Journal of Cardiovascular Prevention & Rehabilitation* 13, no. 5 (2006): 798–804.

using only half the calories of an endurance-training program raised the resting metabolic rates of the test subjects so much that they burned nine times as much fat as the endurance-training group.[6] Another study in the *Journal of Applied Physiology* concluded that interval training enhanced aerobic capacity more efficiently than endurance training.[7] So if you are wondering why there are no "aerobic" or "endurance" exercises in this book, the reason is that the HIIT program develops aerobic capacity and endurance far better than aerobics or endurance exercises, so they aren't needed.

HIIT training increases your fat and carbohydrate metabolism, so you burn fat faster even while you sleep.[8, 9] It is more than four times as efficient at developing athletic capacity than endurance training.[10] It is more cardioprotective,[11] and it develops aerobic capacity even better than aerobic exercise.[12]

If you have ever been a bodybuilder or a competitive weight lifter, you may be surprised to discover that "going heavy" is not necessary to build muscle and functional strength. It may indeed

[6] A. Tremblay, J. A. Simoneau, and C. Bouchard, "Impact of Exercise Intensity on Body Fatness and Skeletal Muscle Metabolism," *Metabolism* 43, no. 7 (1994): 814–18.

[7] K. A. Burgomaster, G. J. Heigenhauser, and M. J. Gibala, "Effect of Short-term Sprint Interval Training on Human Skeletal Muscle Carbohydrate Metabolism During Exercise and Time-Trial Performance," *Journal of Applied Physiology* 100, no. 6 (2006): 2041–47.

[8] C. G. Perry *et al.*, "High-Intensity Aerobic Interval Training Increases Fat and Carbohydrate Metabolic Capacities in Human Skeletal Muscle," *Applied Physiology, Nutrition, and Metabolism* 33, no. 6 (2008): 1112–23.

[9] J. L. Talanian *et al.*, "Two Weeks of High-Intensity Aerobic Interval Training Increases the Capacity for Fat Oxidation During Exercise in Women," *Journal of Applied Physiology* 102, no. 4 (2007): 1439–47.

[10] M. J. Gibala *et al.*, "Short-Term Sprint Interval Versus Traditional Endurance Training: Similar Initial Adaptations in Human Skeletal Muscle and Exercise Performance," *Journal of Physiology* 575, pt. 3 (2006): 901–11.

[11] U. Wisløff *et al.*, "Superior Cardiovascular Effect of Aerobic Interval Training Versus Moderate Continuous Training in Heart Failure Patients: A Randomized Study," *Circulation* 115, no. 24 (2007): 3086–94.

[12] A. M. McManus *et al.*, "Improving Aerobic Power in Primary School Boys: A Comparison of Continuous and Interval Training," *International Journal of Sports Medicine* 26, no. 9 (2005): 781–86.

be necessary for specialized disciplines, but in terms of triggering muscle growth, a HIIT program using multiple sets of 30 percent $R_{max}$ to failure generated *double* the hypertrophy of a single set of 80 percent $R_{max}$ to failure. ($R_{max}$ is the maximum amount of weight a person can lift for one repetition. "Failure" means doing the particular exercise until you cannot do it any further.)[13]

So we have rediscovered the caveman way, renamed it "HIIT," and discovered that it is the most amazing training technique ever. This is, of course, not surprising, as it is precisely how our bodies were designed.

## Cross-Training

Cavemen had well-rounded athletic abilities because the demands of their environment required just about everything that a human being can do. They had to run, jump, lift, carry, throw, climb, and club territorial trespassers. In other words, they were athletic generalists.[14] Though it is possible to specialize in throwing the javelin or simply having large muscles, the best approach for general health is to train the entire body to develop strength, flexibility, endurance, and balance.

Furthermore, all of their strength was functional strength. That is, all of the strength they developed was useful. If you use a weight machine at the gym that locks all of your motion into a single plane without wobble and you develop the ability to lift 100 lbs on that machine, you may be shocked to discover that you can't lift or control 100 lbs using a similar movement in real life. A cross-training type of program concentrates on movements that use multiple joints without outside supports so that all of your muscles and connective tissues have to develop together. In the

---

[13] C. J. Mitchell *et al.*, "Resistance Exercise Load Does Not Determine Training-Mediated Hypertrophic Gains in Young Men," *Journal of Applied Physiology* 113, no. 1 (2012): 71–77.

[14] L. Cordain and J. Friel, eds., *The Paleo Diet for Athletes: A Nutritional Formula for Peak Athletic Performance* (New York: Rodale Books, 2005).

final analysis, the strength and endurance you develop that way will be much more useful in real life.

## Program Overview

This is likely the simplest resistance exercise program in existence. There are five types of exercise in this program: core, upper body push, upper body pull, lower body, and whole body.

For each workout, choose one core exercise that you do before the interval training. For the interval training you choose one push exercise, one pull exercise, and one of *either* lower-body or whole-body exercises. So you choose a total of four exercises for each workout. For complete development, you should change the exercises for each workout.

Each workout consists of:

- At least one of the proprioception and balance exercises from chapter 14
- A selection of three or more dynamic stretches from chapter 15
- One core exercise done continuously until just before failure or for one minute, whichever comes first
- Three to five interval training super sets made up of:
- Upper body push for thirty seconds, rest for thirty seconds
- Upper body pull for thirty seconds, rest for thirty seconds
- Lower body or whole-body for thirty seconds, rest for thirty seconds
- A selection of any five static stretches from chapter 15, based on what you feel needs to be stretched.

Once you have worked up to full workouts, if you are doing this right, when you're done you'll sound like you are hyperventilating as you gasp for precious oxygen, your legs will be shaking, your fine motor skills will be toast, and you'll have to keep telling anyone else in the house with you not to call an ambulance. If you flounce away from your workout as though nothing has happened, then you aren't doing it right.

I am exaggerating but only slightly. These workouts are intended to be very physically demanding, which means they will be difficult and painful, which means they will be psychologically challenging as well. If you aren't used to pushing yourself, you may need to get acclimated to the movements and routine before you jump in.

## Intensity Is the Key

For each set, each interval, and each workout . . . intensity is the key. Think of intensity as the *total work performed in a given amount of time.* The intensity of each instance of an exercise in the superset is adjusted such that it is done nearly to failure. Not quite to failure, but nearly so. For example, your first set of push-ups might be done with your feet on a chair to make them more difficult, whereas your third set might be done with your hands on stair steps to make them easier. Your last repetition should be difficult, but you shouldn't work quite to the point where you couldn't possibly do another.

In a weight lifting scenario, these would be called "drop sets," in which a bit of weight is removed from the barbell for successive sets. But since these movements are done using body weight, you vary the intensity by changing the angles, doing the exercises more slowly, and resting a bit between repetitions and similar adaptations.

What the HIIT technique combined with body weight resistance will accomplish is a progressive adaptation of your body to ever greater total workloads. Because there is a wide variety of angles and exercises, over time you'll build total-body fitness with measurable increases in muscular strength, endurance, cardiovascular fitness, flexibility, and balance. You can call this whole-body athleticism.

I am going to give some concrete examples to illustrate how to apply intensity in practice. When I do a standard push-up, my arms are lifting a weight of 135 lbs. Pretend that I can only do one push-up in a thirty-second time frame, so the total work I do is to lift 135 lbs. If I do an inclined push-up by putting my hands on a stable chair, my arms are instead lifting 90 lbs. Pretend that I can do ten inclined push-ups within thirty seconds, so the total amount of work I have performed is 90 lbs times ten repetitions for a total of 900 lbs. Which is going to develop my body's functional capacity to a higher degree? The answer is obvious: the incline push-ups.

Your goal is to change the intensity such that, in each set, you are getting the maximum amount of work performed during that set and working until the very end of the allocated time. It is entirely okay to "cheat." Pretend that I can do only three standard push-ups without rest and that each one takes me two seconds to perform. Then I should do three push-ups, drop one of my knees to the floor to rest for the space of three breaths, then bring my knee back up into position and do three more. You can break it up any way you want: five push-ups then rest, three push-ups then rest, two push-ups then rest, etc. Just keep going for the entire thirty seconds.

Looking at what I just described, within thirty seconds, even if I couldn't blast out ten push-ups all at once, by resting judiciously I'd still be able to do ten push-ups within thirty seconds, giving me 1,350 lbs of work during that time frame.

You will find that by focusing on intensity, that is, by focusing on the greatest amount of work you can do within a given time frame, you will achieve the greatest gains. Before you know it, you'll be doing more push-ups than you thought possible in thirty seconds and even increasing the intensity by doing decline push-ups with your feet up on a bench.

Obviously, there is a point of diminishing returns in terms of decreasing the effort required for an individual repetition of a given exercise. If I were to lie on a bench pressing a ten-pound weight thirty times in thirty seconds, it would get me nowhere. Adjust the effort so that the last repetition within the thirty-second time frame is difficult but not impossible, and you will have hit the sweet spot.

## Intensity and the Sedentary Individual

As you may have noticed from the above example, what exactly constitutes "intense" will vary from person to person, exercise to exercise, and day to day. I designed this program so that it can be performed in the privacy of your own home. You're not competing against anyone but yourself. Maybe instead of a push-up, the exercise will be sufficiently intense if you just push yourself off a wall or the back of a couch. Maybe an inverted row isn't within your reach right now. If that's the case, set up your suspension trainer, lean back a couple of feet while holding the handles, and pull yourself upright.

The same goes for things like box jumps. In the illustrations of the exercise, a young lady easily hops up onto an eighteen-inch bench. Especially if you are seriously overweight or elderly, that might not be possible or wise. If you can't jump up onto the box, then step up onto it instead.

If you can't do a prescribed exercise, then do a less difficult version of the same exercise or substitute an exercise from the same category that you can do. The key is to reach the maximum intensity within your current capacity. Don't worry about what other people are doing. Instead, just stick with it, and you will see results.

Negative reps are another useful technique. Pretend, for example, that you can't do even a single pull-up—or maybe you can do one pull-up but not enough to fill a thirty-second training interval. Don't sweat it. Instead, for your reps, jump up with your chin already over the bar, and let yourself down slowly. Pretend you can't do push-ups. Start off in a high push-up position, then just let yourself down slowly even if you can't push yourself back up. Because of the tension needed to control your descent, you will eventually build the muscles you need to perform the exercises normally.

You can also do negative reps with other exercises. The key is do what you can even if you can't do an exercise or can't do many reps, then do negative reps, use assistance, or switch to a less tax-ing version. Whatever you do, keep up the workout.

You can also use assisting mechanisms. For example, there are a couple of companies that make large resistance bands that attach to a pull-up bar and to your feet that provide as much as 50 lbs of assistance. Then, as you get stronger, you remove the bands. This works quite well!

Don't take what I am saying here as an excuse to loaf. There is no excuse for loafing. Rather, what I am saying is to work to the *maximum of your individual capacity,* whatever that capacity may be. Over time, your capacity *will* increase. Dramatically.

## Discomfort and Soreness

Unaccustomed exercise means pushing beyond your current limits. When you do this, your body breaks down muscle. The result is pain during an exercise and soreness for maybe even days afterwards. This is normal. During the rest between sessions, your body rebuilds the muscles stronger than they were before. It will also build stronger bones and stronger ligaments.

During unaccustomed exercise, there is a buildup of lactic acid in your muscles, and this accumulation of lactic acid creates a very distinctly uncomfortable burning feeling. Initially, your cells aren't able to dispose of the lactic acid very efficiently, so it doesn't take much effort for the burning to start. But as you get used to greater and greater levels of effort, your body will adapt to become more efficient at disposing the lactic acid.

Soreness is caused by a combination of indisposed lactic acid and damage to muscle cells. These become internally inflamed while being repaired. If you have been a couch potato all your life, this will be unpleasant. You may even find it hard to walk for the first few days after your first few truly intense workouts. If you are already following a modern caveman diet, your diet is rich in anti-oxidants (for scavenging the free radicals) and anti-inflammatory omega-3 fats, so you'll be fine.

All of the foregoing that I am describing is perfectly normal and healthy. I'm letting you know what to expect. Just stick with it. Over time, your body will adapt, and it will take more and more effort to make your muscles burn or to make you sore. But initially, if you are unaccustomed to hard physical effort, you are going to have to adopt an indomitable spirit and learn to love the burning, soreness, and gasping for breath like a fish out of water.

Physical fitness is just like anything else in life that can't be granted by legislation: You will only get out of it what you put into it. And the more of yourself you put into it, the greater the rewards.

## Neurological Recruitment

There are a couple of aspects to practical strength that are inter-related. So far, I have mostly been discussing muscular adaptations, but there are neurological adaptations as well. Your practical strength is a combination of both your absolute muscular strength *and* how much of that strength your nervous system knows how to use.

If you aren't used to employing your muscles intensely, your neurological system doesn't yet know how to recruit the maximum number of muscle fibers. It's a skill that takes practice, but your nervous system learns quickly and will adapt far more quickly than your muscles.

The practical consequence of this is that you will likely see major increases in practical strength within just a couple of weeks. These increases are almost totally the result of your nervous system learning how to work more efficiently with your muscles.

Most newcomers see rapid progress that seems to suddenly hit a wall. Don't be discouraged. As long as you keep up the intensity, you will definitely make progress, but it will be slow and steady.

## More Elite Fitness

As you get used to this system of exercise, you can increase your number of supersets from three to five. If, after a while, you find you aren't even breaking a sweat by doing five rounds of intervals, you can increase the intensity even further by gradually lengthening the "on" period of the exercise sets from thirty seconds to any value up to a full sixty seconds. Another excellent technique for increasing intensity is to perform exercises extremely slowly to maintain muscular tension. How long can you hold yourself in a halfway-up push-up or pull-up position?

I am, however, reminded of a conversation I had with a young man who told me he had sprinted for ten minutes. No, he didn't. If he thinks he sprinted for ten minutes, then he has no conception of what it means to sprint. The longest distance that can conceivably be truly sprinted in all-out effort is a quarter of a mile, and high school athletes complete that distance in *less than a minute.*

If you can do a given exercise for more than sixty seconds continuously, then you need to increase its level of difficulty in some way. Do your push-ups with a kid sitting on your back. Do your pull-ups while wearing a weight vest. Do your box jumps at a greater height while carrying a Volkswagen. (I'm kidding about carrying a Volkswagen, but you get the idea.)

For most people who are interested in excellent fitness rather than *elite* fitness, the program described here will take them well beyond their wildest dreams of how strong, fast, and capable they ever thought they could be. But for those aspiring to elite levels of fitness, this program is insufficient for a couple of reasons.

The first reason is that elite fitness is as much a matter of skill building as fitness, and skill building is beyond the scope of this particular program.

The second reason is that I designed this as a "no excuses" program. With the exception of the shuttle run and sprinting, everything in this program can be done in a 6 ft. x 6 ft. square of space in a rented apartment and with an investment of less than $100 in equipment. All you absolutely need is a pull-up bar and a cheap suspension trainer, though the kettlebell, exercise ball, and medicine ball will certainly help. But how many people live in a place where they can drop a set of barbells from overhead onto their floor? Or hang a fifteen-foot climbing rope or a set of gymnastics rings from the ceiling?

Once someone is ready for elite levels of fitness, this person is ready to graduate from this basic caveman fitness program into something else!

## Men Versus Women

Other than the difference in the weight of kettlebells and medicine balls recommended (see the next section) there is no difference in the program for men and women. Because this is predominantly a body weight HIIT program, it automatically adapts to each individual without regard to sex, age, or any other factor.

There were female cavemen as well, and they still had to forage and outrun threats to survive. Women who couldn't escape saber-toothed tigers didn't survive to make babies.

## Equipment Needed

The primary equipment you need is your own body, but you will also need a few items that will be used to simulate items present in the natural world to make the most of your program. Individually, none of this equipment is particularly expensive, so if you spread it out over a couple of months, it shouldn't break the bank. This gear is certainly less expensive than a membership at most gyms.

*Disclaimer: I have no financial interest in any of the products I mention here, and nobody has paid me for an endorsement.*

• *Doorjamb pull-up bar:* I have two types of pull-up bars, the Perfect Pullup and the Perfect MultiGym. The Perfect Multigym is better for doing pull-ups, because it stands out away from the door so you don't bump your head when pulling your chin above the bar. The Perfect Pullup is better for inverted rows and as a platform for hanging ab straps for doing hanging knee raises and similar exercises. If you must get only one, go for the MultiGym because you can always use your suspension trainer for inverted rows. (Inverted rows are an exercise described later.)

- *Ab straps:* Ab straps allow you to hang from a pull-up bar without straining your shoulders so you can do hanging knee raises and hanging leg raises. These aren't absolutely necessary, but you may find them helpful.

- *Pull-up assist:* This is optional. If you aren't strong enough to do pull-ups yet, you can do negative reps until you gain the strength. The pull-up assist is a device made with resistance bands that ties onto the pull-up bar, and you place one of your feet in it. You can adjust how much assistance it provides by adding or removing resistance bands as you gradually gain strength.

- *Suspension trainer:* There are several varieties of this with a wide range of prices. I use the Trainer In a Bag by WOSS Enterprises for $35, which works great, but many other models are available. If price is no object, you can even spend $250 on a TRX system. You really *do* need a suspension trainer because a suspension trainer gives you the ability to vary the resistance of pushing and pulling exercises over a wide range simply by adjusting the length of the trainer or the position of your feet.

- *Kettlebell:* You need only one. If you are a man, get one that weighs 25–35 lbs. If you are a woman, get one that weighs 15–20 lbs. You want a one-piece kettlebell made of iron with a handle large enough that you can grab it with both hands without your hands touching. This is used to train your whole body rather than as a test of strength. If you are tight on cash, you can skip this until further along in your training.

- *Interval timer:* You can download interval timer apps for smart phones for free. I don't like to use my phone while working out, because I don't want to be interrupted, so I use a Gym Boss timer instead. Many models of timers are available, but be sure to use one specifically intended for interval training.

- *Swiss ball:* Swiss balls may be called fitness balls, gym balls, or stability balls. You want a 55 cm or 65 cm model (between

21 in. and 25 in.) depending on your height. You will be using this for stretching. It can also double as a chair because its constant requirement for balancing will reduce the back damage that comes from sitting.

- *Medicine ball:* Medicine balls look like slightly oversized soccer balls that have been filled with sand or something else heavy. You'll be using this to build your back and chest through plyometric exercises. If you are a man, get a 14–15 lbs model, and if you are a woman go for about 10 lbs.

## Example Workout, Beginner

| | |
|---|---|
| *Dynamic Stretches:* | Roll and Reach, Table, Push-up Crawl to Stand, Knee Circles, Straight Leg Pendulum |
| *Core Exercise:* | Straight-Leg Sit-Ups, for 1 minute or until you can't do anymore (whichever comes first) |
| *Three Super Sets:* | Incline Push-Ups for 30 seconds, rest for 30 seconds |
| | Easy Rope Climb for 30 seconds, rest for 30 seconds |
| | Lunges for 30 seconds, rest 30 seconds |
| *Static Stretches:* | Arm Across, Chest Expansion, Cobra |

## Example Workout, Intermediate

| | |
|---|---|
| *Dynamic Stretches:* | Windmills, Knee Circles, Cariocas, Push-Up Crawl to Stand |
| *Core Exercise:* | Plank, for 1 minute or until you can't do anymore (whichever comes first) |
| *Four Super Sets:* | Push-ups for 30 seconds, rest for 30 seconds |
| | Inverted Row for 30 seconds, rest for 30 seconds |

|  |  |
|---|---|
|  | Squats for 30 seconds, rest for 30 seconds |
| *Static Stretches:* | Prone Hamstring Stretch, Prone Gluteus Stretch, Bridging, Bear Awakens in Spring |

## Example Workout, Advanced

|  |  |
|---|---|
| *Dynamic Stretches:* | Windmills, Knee to Chest Walk, Heel Walk, Cariocas, Straight Leg Pendulum |
| *Core Exercise:* | Hanging Knee Raises, for 1 minute or until you can't do anymore (whichever comes first) |
| *Five Super Sets:* | Tricep Push Downs 60 seconds, rest for 30 seconds |
|  | Pull-Ups for 60 seconds, rest for 30 seconds |
|  | Box Jumps for 60 seconds, rest for 30 seconds |
| *Static Stretches:* | Chest Expansion, Cobra, Elbow Push, Buddha Sleeping on Mountain |

The rest in between intervals is an active rest. Walk around, skip, jog, or do whatever else works for you, but do not sit down, lay down, or bend over with your hands resting on your knees.

## Variety, Variety, Variety!

The example workouts are just that: examples. They give you an idea of the structure of a workout, but it's your job to make your own. The key is to mix in variety. If you do three workouts this week, you should use three different core exercises, three different pushing exercises, three different pulling exercises, and three different lower-body/whole-body exercises.

Likewise, I don't know you, and I don't know your capacities or limitations. It's your job to scale this so that it is within your abilities but at the same time stretches you so that every set ends at a level of difficulty that approaches but doesn't quite reach failure.

## Pushing Exercises
### *Push-Up*

The push-up is the king of all exercises. Done properly, it builds your arms, chest, shoulders, and core. Push-ups can be done in a variety of ways to make them easier or harder or to concentrate effort on different muscle groups. What I'm describing here is the standard push-up. If it is too difficult, don't sweat it—just do incline push-ups instead until you are strong enough for the regular kind.

The starting position for a push-up is most easily attained by lying facedown on the floor and putting your palms on the floor so that the tips of your fingers are even with the tops of your shoulders. Keeping your feet close together and your back straight throughout the movement (you should be able to draw a straight line through your shoulders, hips, and feet), push yourself up. Now you are in a perfect starting position.

Each repetition consists of lowering your chest to the floor (but not quite touching) under control and then pushing yourself back up to the starting position while keeping your body rigid.

To put more emphasis on your chest, spread out your hands a little. To put more emphasis on your triceps (the back of your arms), bring your hands more toward the center of your chest.

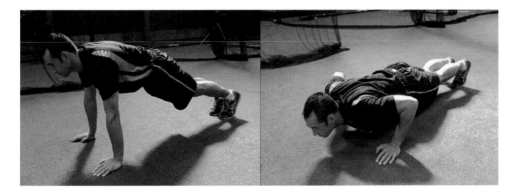

### *Incline Push-Up*
It used to be common to have people who couldn't perform a standard push-up to instruct them to use their knees rather than

their toes as a pivot. The problem is that doing push-ups from the knees negates a lot of the benefit that push-ups give the core. A better option, then, is the incline push-up.

Incline push-ups are performed just like standard push-ups, except the hands are placed on an object that is higher than the floor. This changes the angle and in so doing decreases the amount of weight that has to be lifted. In a standard push-up, you are lifting between 70 and 75 percent of your body weight. So if you weigh 184 lbs, you are lifting about 134 lbs. The higher up you place your hands, the more weight is transferred to your feet and the less you are lifting with your arms and chest.

You can use a solid object for this such as a set of stairs—starting at a high step and then working progressively to lower steps as you gain strength until you can do standard push-ups. If you don't have stairs available, use your suspension trainer for incline push-ups, and you'll get an enormous boost from building the stabilizer muscles needed to stabilize you in three dimensions. You can vary the resistance by changing the length of the straps and the position of your feet.

Though many people improvise and use kitchen chairs for incline push-ups, please be careful with this because if they slide, you could be injured.

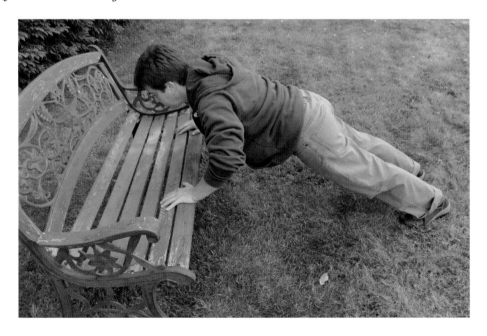

### Decline Push-Up

Just as an incline push-up is used to make push-ups easier, a decline push-up is used to make push-ups harder by elevating the feet rather than the hands. You can elevate your feet by placing them on stairs or a chair. Most suspension trainers also include foot loops, so if you're agile, you can use the suspension trainer to elevate your feet.

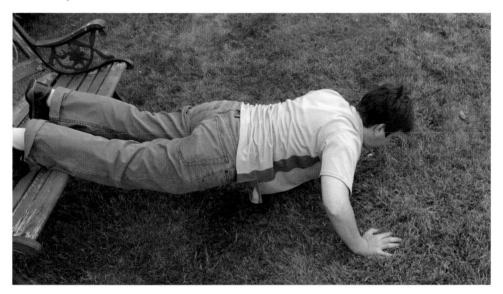

### Medicine Ball Push

Medicine balls are heavy, and mishandling them can result in injury. If you are unused to exercise, wait until you've been doing other pushing exercises for a while and feel ready before using a medicine ball. Also, this exercise can't be done in a typical home, so do it outside or in a gym.

Hold the medicine ball to your chest, then explosively thrust it

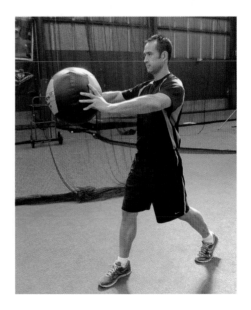

outward away from you as hard as you can. Go get the ball, then do it again. It is important when doing this exercise to keep your elbows rigged into your sides and push straight out.

## Falling Push-up

Falling push-ups are advanced plyometric movements that depend on a good sense of timing and proprioception as well as strength in order to perform them without injury. After you've been working out for a while and are confident, you can try this out. It's an excellent movement for building explosive power.

Get set up as though you were going to do incline push-ups. From a standing position, fall straight-bodied toward the object you'll be using. Catch yourself with your hands so your head doesn't hit the object, cushioning your fall. Then immediately thrust yourself backward. Repeat.

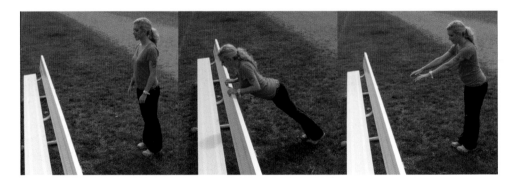

## Military Press

The military press is a pushing movement that works primarily the shoulders. It can be done in both a basic and an advanced method. The basic method is to stand tall, then bend at the waist and put your hands on the floor a comfortable distance (two to four feet) in front of your feet. Execute the movement by using your arms to gently lower yourself until your head touches the floor and then pushing yourself back up. The basic form of this movement has you lifting between 50 and 55 percent of your bodyweight.

If this is insufficiently challenging as you become fitter, you can go all the way up to your full body weight by using a suspension trainer. From a high push-up position, hook your feet in the loops of your suspension trainer as though you were doing decline push-ups. Then, walk backward on your hands, keeping your body straight as your feet go higher into the air. The higher your feet are and the more your body assumes a straight up and down position, the more of your weight will be lifted by your arms.

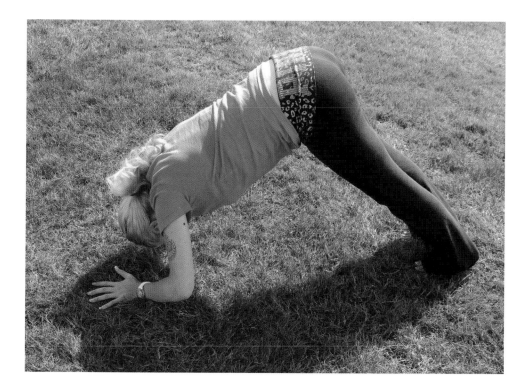

## Tricep Dip

Though tricep dips can be performed as an isolation exercise for just one muscle group, the body weight variation also works your shoulders. For this exercise I use two short stepladders that I am sure won't slide or tip.

Set the ladders a comfortable distance apart so you can fit between them. Using your heels as a fulcrum and keeping your legs straight and horizontal and your torso vertical, use your hands placed palm down on the chairs to push yourself up. Then let yourself back down and repeat.

If this movement is too difficult, you can make it easier by bending your knees so that your feet are flat on the floor, your knees are at a ninety-degree angle, and your torso is vertical.

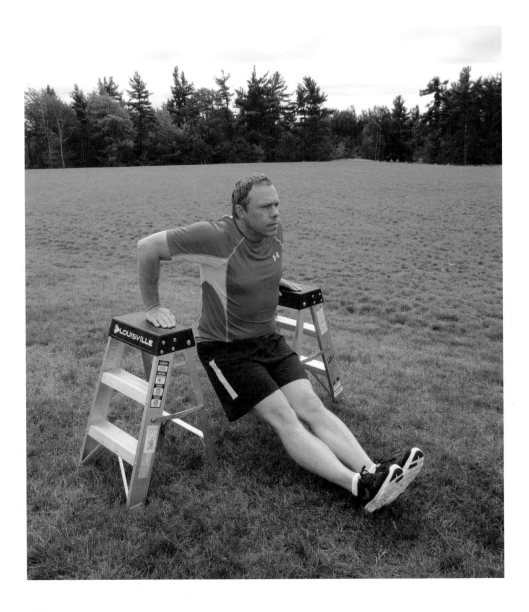

## Pulling Exercises

### Medicine Ball Throw and Catch

Though this isn't an obvious pulling exercise, it works as a plyometric pull because of the muscles it stretches as you catch the ball. Medicine balls are heavy. A ball weighing several pounds falling on your head could hurt or kill you. You should wait to attempt this exercise until you are confident in your hand-eye coordination and your proprioception is solid.

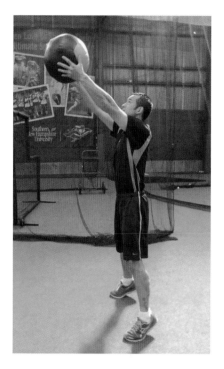

Cradle the medicine ball in your hands. Using your whole body, hurl it straight up in the air. Position yourself to catch it by cradling it, then catch the ball as it falls. If you look like you'll miss, just step back away from the ball so you don't get hurt. Once you get good at this, it will become one of your all-time favorite exercises.

### Inverted Row

Use your suspension trainer (or a low bar if you have one), setting the handles at about waist height. (You may need to experiment because everyone's body is a bit different.) Lie on the floor faceup under the handles. Keeping your body straight and pivoting on your heels, grab the handles and pull yourself up until the handles are even with your chest, and then let yourself back down.

If this is too difficult at first, just bend your knees and put your feet flat on the floor so that your knees will be the pivot point. You can vary the resistance by changing the angle of your knees and the placement of your feet.

If you are not yet strong enough for pull-ups, this is a great exercise to start building your back. Regardless, even if you are doing pull-ups aplenty, you shouldn't ignore this exercise, because it hits your muscles at different angles.

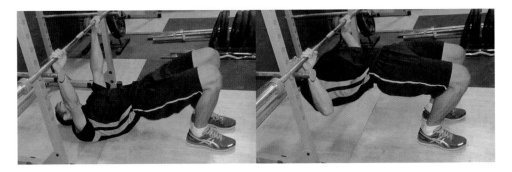

## *Pull-Up*

If the push-up is the king of exercises, the pull-up is next in line for the throne. The trouble is that most people can't do even one pull-up, so they are stuck in a quandary of wondering how to improve at something they can't do at all. First I'll describe how to do a pull-up, and then I'll go into the various ways of working up to your first full pull-up.

Jump up and put your hands on the bar, about shoulder-width apart and palms facing out. (You can also do palms facing inward, which is called a chin-up. Either direction is fine.) Let your body stop swinging, then pull down on your hands until your chin is above the bar, then let yourself back down. The key to this is to apply pressure smoothly. I've known people who thought they couldn't do a pull-up when they really could but they were using jerking motions rather than applying steady pressure. Also, pay attention to the fact that it works better when your elbows stay in front of you rather than in a plane with your body like wings. Over time, you'll be able to do it both ways.

If you can't do a pull-up, you can work your way up to it. First, concentrate on your inverted rows for a while. Once you can do twenty inverted rows in a row from your heels, you can switch to doing negative-rep pull-ups. To do a negative rep, jump up and allow your momentum to help propel your chin over the bar, then let yourself down slowly. Repeat. Keep doing this with your workouts until you can do ten negative reps in a row. Now, try your first pull up. If you still can't quite do it, just give yourself a little "assist" by standing on something so you don't have to do a full rep. Bring yourself to the top, then bend your knees and go all the way down. Put your feet down to push yourself up and repeat. After you can do ten of these, you'll definitely be able to do full pull-ups!

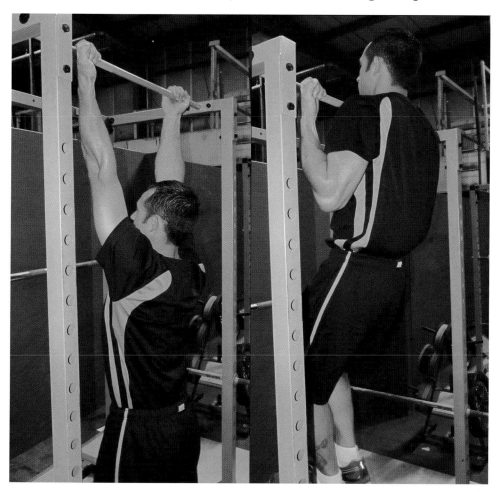

## *Easy Rope Climb*

Tie a nice long (about fifteen feet should be enough) rope that is thick enough that you can grab it easily to your pull-up bar.

Digging your heels into the ground and keeping your body straight, lower yourself to the ground hand over hand. Now, pull yourself back up to a standing position hand over hand.

You can find rope suitable for this at the big chain home-improvement stores. I use two pieces of ¾ in. nylon rope that I hold together to help build hand strength.

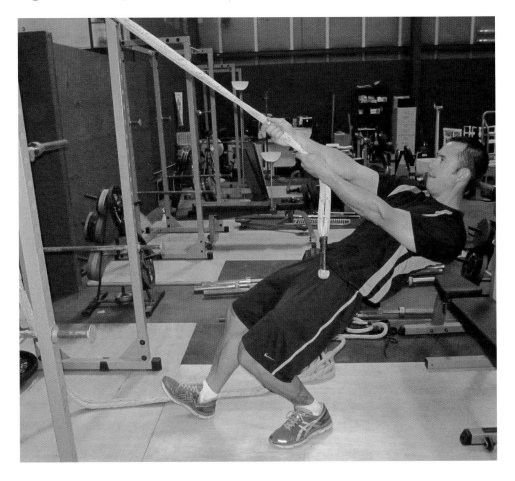

## Lower Body
### *Body Weight Squat*

For some of us, body weight squats are the most fun you can have without getting arrested. It's obvious that they help build your legs and glutes, but it is less obvious that they help you build balance and flexibility.

Stand with your feet shoulder-width apart with your toes pointing *slightly* outward. Hold your arms straight out and palm down. Keeping your back straight or slightly arched back, bend the hips and knees until your thighs are parallel to the floor, then raise yourself back up.

The bodyweight squat is a crucial movement, and there are a couple of fine points about this movement. Make sure that your knees stay over your feet rather than bent inward or outward during this movement. Keep the back straight. (Straight does not mean vertical.) You can go as far down as you want, so long as your heels do not leave the floor.

It's not unusual for people to have difficulty going very deeply into this movement. Simply go as far as you can comfortably, and go further as you improve. There is one stretch I have found useful in teaching proper squat form, called the Chinese Wall Squat. Stand with your feet four inches from a wall, your hands at your side and your feet the proper distance apart for a squat. Now, squat down slowly as far as you can go without any part of you touching the wall. Make sure your knees track properly over your feet. If you add this to your static stretches at the end of your workouts, you'll find that it helps a lot.

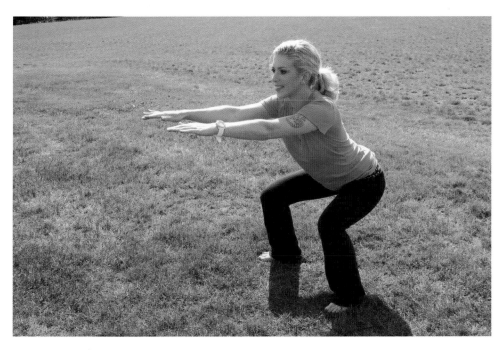

### *Single-Leg Split Squat*

Single-leg split squats are just a body weight squat during which you raise the intensity by using one leg at a time. To perform this exercise, you'll need something to place behind you that is about sixteen inches tall. I use the second step on some stairs in my house, but a step stool will do fine.

Place your device about a foot behind you and slightly left of your center. Step forward about a foot with your right foot, and rest your left instep on the device so you are standing balanced on your right foot. Now, lower yourself on your right leg until your thigh is parallel to the ground, then lift yourself back up. Do all the repetitions for one side before switching to the other.

This exercise will challenge your balance a bit while building impressive functional strength.

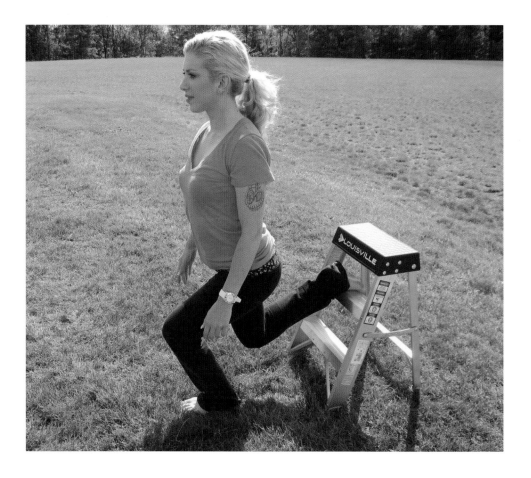

## Lunges

Lunges are a great exercise for building explosive power in your legs. Stand tall with your hands relaxed. Step forward with your right leg far enough that your shin is straight up and down and your thigh is nearly parallel to the floor. It is normal for your left knee to bend and come close to the floor when you do this, but don't step outward so far that you bang your knee. Then, push off of your right leg hard enough that you return to your starting position. Repeat with your left leg.

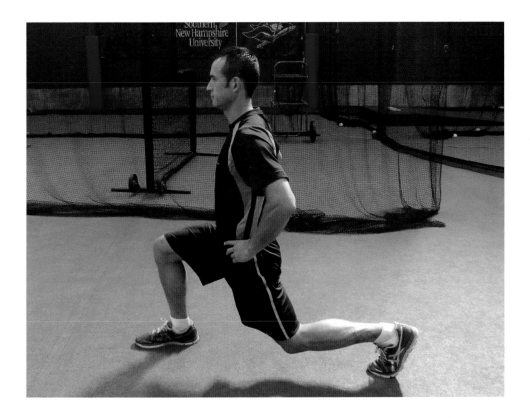

## Side Lunges

Side lunges really work your hips and inner thighs while improving your hip flexibility. Stand tall with your hands relaxed at your waist. Step out to the right with your right leg far enough that your shin is straight up and down and your thigh is nearly parallel with the floor. Now, push off your right leg so that you return to your starting position. Do all of your reps on the right leg, then switch and repeat using your left leg. This exercise can be hard on your knees, so if you have bad knees, skip it.

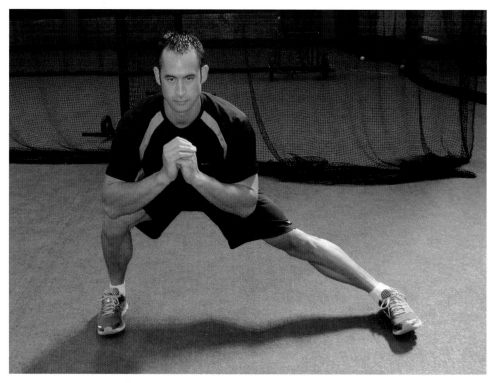

## Whole Body
### *Burpees*

Despite the funny name, this is a powerful whole-body exercise. Burpees will transform you into a lean, mean caveman machine!

Stand with your feet slightly more than shoulder-width apart, squat down, and put both of your hands on the floor. Thrust out your legs to assume a high push-up position. Execute a push-up. Once you return to the high push-up position, bring your legs back under your body, then jump up into the air with your hands outstretched reaching for the sky. Execute the various phases of this exercise smoothly.

As you can see, this is a whole-body workout all by itself, which is why it is so popular with the military. If you aren't quite ready for this because you can't do push-ups, just incorporate this later, once you've gained strength. There's no rush!

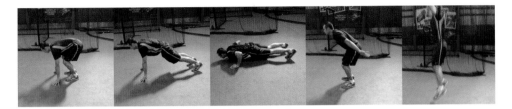

## Box Jumps

This exercise can be dangerous if your proprioception or balance is off. If you aren't confident, wait until you've rebuilt them for a while before attempting to do box jumps.

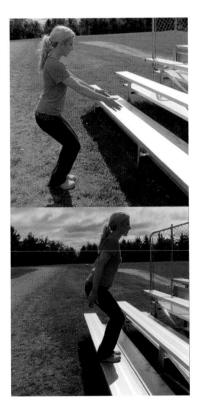

Though elite athletes will do box jumps onto boxes three or four feet high, that is unnecessary for our current goals (though if you want to use higher boxes as you gain fitness that's totally fine!). I use an eighteen-inch step stool with a solid base. The solid base and stability are important! Don't try to jump up onto something that may shift, wobble, or break. You can even use the first or second step on a set of concrete stairs if you have some.

Stand twelve to eighteen inches in front of your box with your knees bent and your feet together. Now, using both feet together, jump up onto the box, then spring back off it backwards into your starting position. This movement should be done with perfect control, so only do it until you start losing your form.

### Jumping Jacks

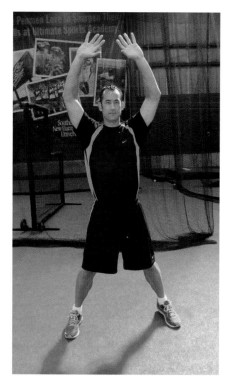

A perennial favorite of drill instructors and physical education coaches since the beginning of time, jumping jacks are an excellent whole-body movement that has stood the test of time. They will work your legs and butt while improving your whole-body flexibility. Plus, jumping jacks are fun!

Stand with your feet together and your hands by your side. Make a slight jump, spreading your legs to form an upside-down V while bringing your hands together to meet above your head. Then make another slight jump bringing your feet back together while returning your hands to your sides. Do it in one smooth motion.

### Kettlebell Swings

Kettlebell swings are a fantastic full-body exercise, but they ought not be attempted until you're very proficient with the body weight squat. Once you can maintain proper form through three sets of squats, you'll be ready for kettlebell swings. There are a few key points that need to be observed with kettlebell swings, some obvious and others subtler.

A kettlebell is a heavy piece of iron. Even a relatively light 25 lbs. kettlebell weighs three times as much as a sledgehammer. If it lands on someone's foot or hits a person on the head, it will be a negatively life-altering experience at best. When swinging a kettlebell, be aware of your surroundings and the kettlebell's trajectory! If you lose control of the kettlebell, step away from its path.

When using the kettlebell, keep your spine straight at all times. Do not round your back or your shoulders! Keep your shoulders firmly back in their sockets, and lock out your elbows. When you are done using the kettlebell, use a static stretch such as the Cobra to keep your back bent backwards for a little while. Failure to observe these precautions *will* result in maladies such as lower back pain, tennis elbow, and torn rotator cuffs.

Casual observation of kettlebell swings could lead you to believe that they are powered primarily by the arms and upper body strength when nothing could be further from the truth. In fact, the arms and hands are acting more like the rope on a tire swing, and it is an explosive force from your hips that generates the power to push the swing. Little if any upper body strength is used. If you find yourself trying to muscle the kettlebell, you are doing it wrong.

The movement of a kettlebell swing is essentially a squat. When you go from the squatting to standing position, you do so with sufficient snap so that the force of your pelvis against your forearms propels the kettlebell into the air.

Start in a low squat position with the kettlebell resting on the ground between your feet. Grab the kettlebell's handle with both hands using an overhand grip, raising up to a half-squat position with the kettlebell hanging loosely between your legs. Maintain a straight back! (Straight is not vertical.) Give the kettlebell a slight swing backwards between your legs as though you were hiking a football, then drive your feet straight into the floor as you straighten your hips explosively as though you were going to jump into the air, except keep your feet on the ground and focus that force through your pelvis into your forearms.

The kettlebell will be propelled into the air at the ends of your arms. Toward the top of its arc (which should be at chest or eye level), it will become weightless before it starts falling. As it descends, use your arms (keeping your elbows locked and shoulders in the sockets) to guide the arc of the kettlebell back between your legs as you return to your half-squat initial position.

I have included pictures demonstrating the key starting and weightless positions, but if you still find yourself stymied, there are a number of video presentations of kettlebell swings on the Internet. Once you get good at these, they'll quickly become a favorite movement. During the weightless phase, once you are experienced, you can even change from two-handed to one-handed swings or alternate between using just the left or right arm.

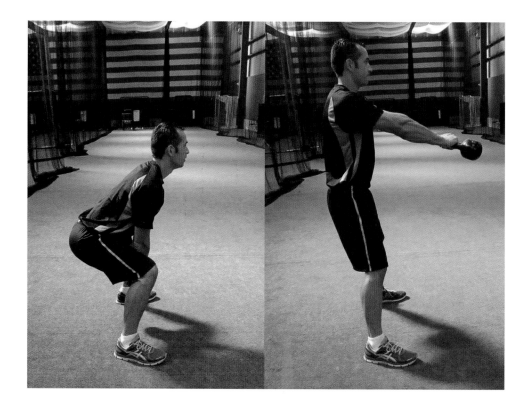

## *Shuttle Run*

The shuttle run was used to test physical fitness in school children and is still part of the President's physical fitness challenge. This is a wonderful exercise because you have to run full speed, stop quickly, and bend. This is an outdoor exercise unless you have a gym with lots of free floor space at your disposal.

Make two lines on the ground thirty feet apart. Place two objects (I use a garden trowel, but anything small and portable will do) behind one of the lines. Go stand behind the other line. Now, run as fast as you can, grab one of the objects, run back, and place it where you were standing, then turn around and run to get the other object and bring it back, crossing your finish line at full speed.

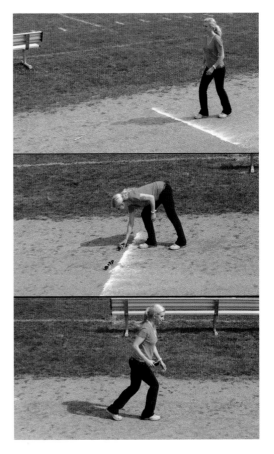

## Sprints

Sprints are the ultimate metabolic enhancer bar none. They are exactly what they sound like—you run as fast as you possibly can for a set short distance. Though this seems like it is primarily a leg exercise, every muscle in your body—even the small muscles between your ribs—comes into play. You'll need to do sprints outdoors, though certain models of treadmills can allow you to sprint safely.

To do HIIT with sprints, you sprint the distance, turn around and walk back, then do it again.

Sprinting is extremely strenuous and something you'll need to work up to if you haven't done it since childhood. If you don't take your time and work up to it, you will pull hamstrings and do all sorts of damage.

Obviously, doing all the other parts of this program will help you prepare, but you need other preparation as well. I do my work at a local high school track, and most towns have such a place available and accessible. If you don't, you can use what I call the "driveway method."

A high school track is 440 yards in circumference. The straightaways are 110 yards, and the curves are 110 yards. Walk completely around the track once taking long strides. Then, on your second lap, stretch out your legs and do a gentle run (not a jog, not a sprint, but a *run*) along the straightaways, and walk around the curves. Do this for two more laps. Do this workout once a week for a few weeks, gradually increasing the speed on the straightaways until you are sprinting them.

The driveway method is something I devised while living in a ridiculously congested suburb. You walk the distance of the yards and run across the driveways and cross streets. Because you can't effectively measure distance, do it for twelve minutes. Just as with using the high school track, gradually increase the speeds of the running portion until you can sprint.

Once you've worked up to sprinting, you'll notice something interesting about your body: It looks fabulous!

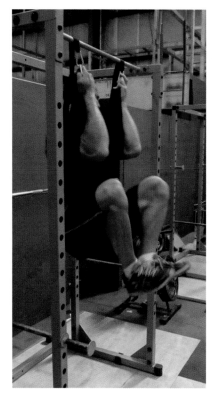

## Core

### *Hanging Knee Raise*

Most of the exercises in this program work your core (abs, sides, and lower back) indirectly and, done over time, will result in adequate abdominal development. The primary reason most folks don't have defined abs is a layer of fat that obscures them. All the core exercises in the world won't give defined abs if there's a layer of fat. So these core exercises are intended more for rounding out body development. Given a caveman diet and fitness program, as the fat disappears, your abs will come out.

Though you can do this exercise while hanging from a pull-up bar (and when you are strong enough, I would encourage that), it is most easily done using ab straps. Ab straps allow you to rest your upper arms in the straps, removing stress from your arms so they aren't a limiting factor in working your abs.

Hang from the bar with your body straight. Raise your knees toward your chest, using your abdominal muscles to bring your knees as close to your elbows as you can. Then slowly return to the starting position.

Do these to near failure or until you can go a minute without stopping.

### Straight-Leg Sit-Up

Lie flat on your back with your arms outstretched along the floor above your head. Keeping your hands along the floor, slowly sit up until you can touch your toes with your fingers, then slowly return to the starting position and repeat.

Do these continuously for a full minute or until you feel like you can do only one more.

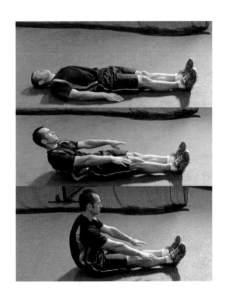

### Crunch

Lie flat on your back with your knees bent and your feet flat on the floor. Cross your hands over your chest. Now, raise your torso until your shoulder blades are no longer touching the floor. When you do this movement, you should be trying to move your body up rather than toward your knees. Return to the starting position and repeat.

Crunches work best at developing your upper abs. You should start off with ten and work your way up to forty or more over time.

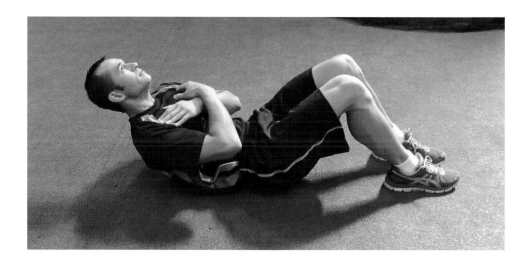

## *Plank*

Starting from a high push-up position, put your forearms on the floor with your palms facing down and your upper arms positioned vertically. Hold your body straight in this position. At first, holding this position for thirty seconds will be challenging but you want to work your way up to two minutes as you make progress.

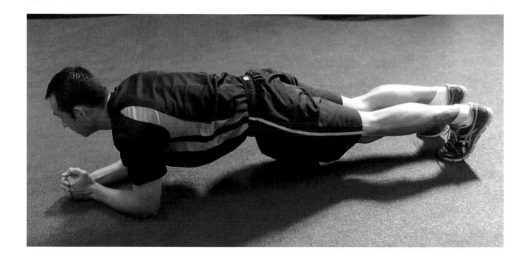

# Chapter 17
## FAQs and Roadblocks

When I started writing this book, I had in mind the dozens or hundreds of questions people had asked me about the diet over time. Consequently, it has been my intention to answer most questions within this book. There are, inevitably, a few straggling questions that don't fit logically within the context of the chapters, so I've reserved those questions for this final chapter.

### If This Diet Is So Great, Why Doesn't My Doctor Recommend It?

Give your doctor a copy of this book, highlighting the hundreds of studies I've cited, and *ask your doctor* why he or she doesn't recommend it. Most likely, because doctors are no different than anyone else in some respects, it is simple adherence to orthodoxy. Sixty years ago doctors recommended smoking. Forty years ago doctors recommended trans fats. Today they recommend soybean oil.

Because I'm not a medical doctor, I recommend that you examine the available data and reach your own conclusions.

### My Aunt Maddie Is 156 Years Old and Eats Spaghetti Every Day

Good for her! Every person has a slightly different set of evolutionary adaptations, and there are some people who are better adapted to certain foods than others. Your aunt is obviously well-adapted to the modern diet.

Everything is a game of odds. Though dietary recommendations and the results of studies are often presented as absolutes, nothing could be further from the truth. There are outliers in every study. I am certain that somewhere there is a person who thrives on drinking soft drinks and gorging on ice cream to the exclusion of all other foods. But what are the odds that *you* are such a person?

What I have presented here is an argument based on statistics and probability. If you dig into the studies I've cited, you'll find that some of them are just pages and pages of statistical analysis. It is statistically likely that you are best adapted for exactly what I have laid down in this book, but a statistical likelihood is *not* a guarantee. I suggest trying what I have laid down religiously for a few months and then honestly assess how you feel. Odds are, you'll be a believer.

## Even After Adopting Caveman Diet, I am Having Autoimmune Problems

Once you have developed an immune response, your body has a memory of that response that can last for many years or even your entire life. This is the entire principle behind vaccination and why it can convey lifetime immunity against a deadly illness.

Not all immune responses last forever. Some will disappear almost immediately once the offending substance has been removed. Some will disappear over a course of weeks or months—sometimes years. And some, as stated, will last the rest of your life. I cannot tell you with certainty which circumstance applies in your case, and nobody else can tell you either. It's a matter of wait and see while doing the best you can not to exacerbate the condition or add new problems.

If you've been following a caveman diet for a year or more and you are still having problems with an autoimmune disease such as arthritis, the one other food group that might yield results if eliminated is nightshade family plants.

The science is not strong on this. Most people gain a lot of benefit from eating plants in this family, such as tomatoes, eggplant, peppers, and so forth. So unlike grains, legumes, and dairy, I don't believe people should utterly eliminate them. If, however, you are having a stubborn autoimmune illness that hasn't responded to the base caveman diet, eliminating nightshades *may* be helpful.

The nightshade family includes a great many deadly poisonous plants, such as datura, belladonna, henbane, and tobacco. But it also includes a large number of foods that we typically eat, including tomatoes, potatoes, eggplant, peppers, tomatillos, ground cherries, and garden huckleberries among others.

Just like grains and legumes, nightshades contain sublethal levels of toxic substances. Eggplant, for example, contains nicotine as well as high levels of histamines, which could easily trigger allergic reactions. All nightshades (plus many plants in other families) contain a poisonous alkaloid called solanine. The levels of both nicotine and solanine in edible nightshades are generally low enough to be a nonissue. You'd have to eat about 100 large tomatoes to get enough nicotine to notice, and you'd have to eat over sixty large potatoes in a single sitting to get enough solanine to cause a reaction.

Plants from the nightshade family also contain a substance called calcitriol, and an excess of this (which can happen in people with compromised kidney function due to a high-carb diet) will cause absorption of excess calcium and deposits of calcium in soft tissue such as joints. This is not a problem for most people, but it can be a problem in some cases.

Tomatine in tomatoes (don't you ever wonder who names these substances?) has been shown to kill a variety of cancer cells, but it can kill normal cells as well.[1] If you already have problems with grain or legume lectins stripping your intestinal mucosa, the tomatine could damage the cells in your intestinal tract, making it easier for foreign proteins to enter the digestive tract and generate immune reactions.

Even though most people don't react adversely, some people become sensitized to nightshade family foods and produce antibodies against them, causing allergic reactions. When this happens, a person consuming them puts the body in a constant state

---

[1] M. Friedman *et al.*, "Tomatine-Containing Green Tomato Extracts Inhibit Growth of Human Breast, Colon, Liver, and Stomach Cancer Cells," *Journal of Agricultural and Food Chemistry* 57, no. 13 (2009): 5727–33.

of inflammation. In addition, the antibodies created could attack other natural body tissues.

So if you are still having autoimmune problems after a year on a cavemen diet, you can try eliminating nightshades. But you should also understand that sometimes the problems caused by a bad diet cannot be completely eliminated by correcting the diet, and the best you can hope for is to not cause new problems.

Another approach worth considering is Functional Diagnostic Nutrition. Very often, even after the source of damage to intestinal mucosa and other systems is removed, the damage remains. Functional Diagnostic Nutrition (no, they haven't paid me for an endorsement) identifies these issues and addresses them holistically.

## I'm Waiting to Quit Smoking Before I Start Working Out

By all means you should quit smoking as soon as you can, but you also shouldn't use one unhealthy habit (smoking) as an excuse to perpetuate an additional unhealthy habit (being sedentary). Don't let the perfect be the enemy of the good. Diet alone is not enough—you must exercise to be healthy!

You may be shocked to learn that many of the world's most elite Olympic athletes, such as Mo Farrah (10 km and 5 km gold medalist) and Jessica Ennis (women's heptathlon gold medalist), are smokers.[2] According to a *Reuters* story about the 2008 Olympics, about 70 percent of Olympic athletes smoke.[3]

Gradually ramp up the intensity of your workouts over a few weeks, and you'll find your decreased lung capacity was mostly caused by bad posture and being sedentary. The decreased stress, depression, and anxiety that you'll experience from getting your exercise will likely even help you stop smoking!

---

[2] "Olympians Blasted for Smoking Outside Stadium," *The Daily Mash*, June 8, 2012.

[3] S. Hardach, "Beijing Smog? I'm Off for a Smoke," *Reuters*, August 6, 2008.

## Eating Out

Believe it or not, with just a few precautions you can eat out even in fast-food restaurants. The big thing you need to watch for is hidden grains, such as flour and corn starch. Chinese food is famous for mixing flour or cornstarch into practically every sauce. But all you have to do is order what you want *without the sauce.* Fried foods are another biggie—not only are they usually coated with grains but also they are then fried in some sort of Frankenstein's monster type of oil.

You'll also find some pretty nasty oils in most salad dressings, but if you get an "olive oil and vinegar" dressing, you should be all set. Beyond that, most condiments are used in sufficiently small quantities as to not be a problem. Barbecue sauce is usually thickened with flour and should be avoided unless you can be assured that it is a gluten-free variety. Some restaurants actually keep gluten-free barbecue sauce available for patrons who request it.

The major fast-food chains (e.g., McDonald's and Wendy's) have grilled-chicken-on-salad options that are pretty reasonable. You can also order a burger without the bun. Many other restaurants offer salads or salad bars, and with "low carb" having caught on, orders of sandwiches without the bun or steaks without the side of rice are quite common and easily accommodated.

## Caretaker Roles and Exercise

Even the modest amount of time needed for your exercise program can be difficult, especially if you are in a role of a caretaker, because people just can't seem to shut off their needs for a whopping thirty-five minutes, and you might even feel guilty for taking that time for yourself. (The classic man or woman who "does too much.")

But here is the thing: You *have* to take care of yourself; otherwise you'll have less and less to give until there is nothing at all left. Your health is at stake here. So tell people to either lead, follow, or get out of the way. Get in your workout, take a quick shower after, and be a better you.

## Making All This Food Takes Too Long!

I covered this in my book *Maximizing Your MiniFarm*. The majority of the time spent cooking hands-on is prep time for getting ingredients out of the refrigerator and so forth. Doubling or tripling the amount cooked only adds a few minutes to your cooking time. So cook extra every time you cook, package entrées and fruit/vegetable courses separately, and pop them in your freezer. Then you'll have delicious caveman cuisine that you can pack for lunch or just zap in the microwave when you get home from work.

Because the time that a large roast, ham, or turkey spends in the oven is mostly time that you can spend doing other things, if you cook a large meat course like this every other weekend and just package it up, pretty soon you'll have more frozen food than you'll know what to do with.

## Sabotage

Another issue you may face is sabotage from loved ones—and this applies to both diet and exercise. An improvement in your physical appearance can heighten insecurities in a mate or cause jealousy in a friend. But it will also make you feel better about yourself, increase your confidence, and increase your effectiveness, and the accompanying increase in fitness will make you more capable overall. You'll even be smarter because increased fitness helps you think better.

What you are doing is for your health and well-being. Though it may have other incidental positive effects, your health and well-being in the long term are the primary drivers, so you don't want to be derailed. At the same time, you don't want your important relationships to suffer.

The first thing I'd recommend is communicating with people in your life. Explain what you are doing and why, and actively enlist their aid if not their participation. Always be open to incorporating loved ones into your positive changes.

If loved ones don't decide to make changes in their lives identical to yours, you have to be okay with that, and you can't berate them. There are many paths to worthy destinations, and everyone is different.

In the final analysis, we're talking about your health and life here. There's no need to be nasty or hurtful, and I certainly don't want to encourage the already epidemic levels of narcissistic "relationship" interaction that are already out there, but your life and quality of life depend on your diet and fitness, so you can't let sabotage succeed.

## This Food Is *Boring*

You can find about five million cookbooks for free or for less than a dollar at yard sales, and nearly all of them give excellent recipes for meats, fruits, and vegetables that are either already caveman-friendly or can be made so with minimal modification. Practically the entire universe of herbs and spices is available for your application, and even if, like me, you aren't the most creative person in the kitchen, there are tons of ideas out there.

One of the most important skills you need to learn is how to cook. I have never understood people neglecting a skill so basic as being able to put food in your belly. Maybe if you are an heir to billions you can afford to neglect such skills, but everyone else needs them. Find some good cookbooks, and pretty soon you'll learn the principles of cooking well enough that you'll never be bored again.

Also, try to think a bit outside the norm. For example, it is typical to thicken sauces and gravies with cornstarch or flour, but you can also use a bit of agar. If you don't want to use agar, you can take dried mushrooms, pulverize them into powder in a blender, and use those. If you have a garden, you can dry okra, pulverize the dehydrated okra in a blender, and use that.

## Get the Bacteria on Your Side

Not being in politics, I don't get paid enough to lie, so you're going to have to settle for the truth: The first couple of weeks on a caveman diet are like going off heroin or crack as your body adjusts. If you have been on the standard American diet, though it isn't obvious, you have some direct and indirect food addictions.

I am using the term "addiction" in an imprecise sense. Drug addictions involve modifications in the number and function of neurotransmitter receptors in the brain and are fixed only when the receptors are repaired in terms of number and function. With the exception of sugar, food addictions aren't quite like that. What you are dealing with instead is damage to your endocrine system and hormonal receptors. So it is a whole-body addiction rather than just a brain addiction.

Your most likely direct addiction is to simple carbohydrates like bread and sugar. Your body is used to periodic jolts of glucose that are only tamped down by doses of insulin. This takes a few weeks to normalize enough for cravings to subside, because creeping insulin resistance has messed up the receptors.

In addition, you likely have a certain amount of leptin resistance. Leptin is a hormone that signals when you are done eating, but the lectins in grains desensitize your leptin receptors so that your body is used to relying on high blood glucose levels to tamp down ghrelin production so you can stop eating. This whole thing is pretty messy, but the end result is that for your first couple of weeks on a caveman diet, you may have a strange hollow feeling in the pit of your stomach as though you are hungry even if you have just personally eaten three bison and an entire apple tree—leaves and all.

Then there are the indirect addictions that have nothing to do with you and everything to do with your gut bacteria. The bacteria in your gut are from hundreds or thousands of species, and the specific species that are living there—and the relative proportions of those species—is a function of your environmental exposures, your specific immune genetics, and the foods you eat. If you eat lots of inulin (found in Jerusalem artichokes) or lots of beans, then your bacterial profile is going to be very different from that of someone who never eats these things.

The bacteria in your gut emit substances that are sensed by the millions of neurons in the gut and that serve to modify your behavior. If your gut bacteria are accustomed to a certain diet and you deprive them of that diet, they are going to object. Therefore, any major change in diet should be preceded by a fast and a purge followed by a probiotic supplement to repopulate your bacteria.

I recommend that you start your fast after dinner on a Friday night, and take a saline laxative (such as Epsom salt in water used according to label directions) before bed. You can drink water and tea, coffee, or herbal tea without any additives the next day and start eating again Saturday evening. Starting with Saturday evening's meal, take a probiotic supplement with each meal for the next week.

You want a *broad spectrum* probiotic. This means more than just acidophilus. You're looking for a supplement with at least seven different species of bacteria. Progressive Labs, Prescript Assist, Primal Defense, and others all make broad spectrum probiotics. You may need to mail-order something because its unlikely that your local grocery store carries what you need.

By reducing the numbers of bacteria that are adapted to your old diet by fasting, purging, and then replenishing with bacteria that will be adapting to your new diet, you'll be priming yourself for success in a difficult endeavor.

## What About Other Supplements?

The only supplements I recommend are vitamin D (5,000 IU daily) if you don't get enough sun, fish oil if you don't get enough fish (but fish is superior), CoQ10 if you are taking statin drugs, and probiotics to help your intestines. There is nothing else that I recommend, because when I have looked at the science objectively, most vitamins give you expensive urine at best and actually predispose a ton of cancers at worst.

There is no pill that is a quick fix for bad diet. You should endeavor to eat a variety of vegetables and fruits daily along with healthy meats and fats. The standard American diet is deficient in practically all vitamins and minerals. But if you follow a caveman diet and look up the nutritional content of what you are eating and add it all up, you'll discover that you are getting anywhere from 400 to 800 percent of the RDA for nearly all vitamins and well over 100 percent for all minerals. The only exception is vitamin D, which you get from sunshine. If you eat a caveman diet, you won't need any supplements.

## Good Luck!

I hope you enjoyed this book and found it informative. I wrote it with the objective in mind of helping people help themselves, and if you are now inspired to make some changes in your diet and lifestyle, my goal has been achieved.

Good luck to you, and I wish the best of health and quality of life for you and your loved ones.

# Index

## A

accelerated aging, 65
acne, 64–67, 73, 74, 92, 177, 189
adaptation, 13–15, 19, 21, 56, 57, 59, 117–118, 169, 248, 253, 257, 285
advanced glycation end products, 105
agave nectar, 175, 176
aging, 65, 71, 77, 85, 105, 107–109, 114, 212
ALA, 84, 85, 88
alcohol, 26, 79, 90, 108, 109, 119, 169–170, 171
allergen, 69
alpha linolenic acid, 84, 85, 88
amaranth, 53
amino acid, 23, 35, 43, 72, 73, 135, 136, 154, 175
amylase, 41, 46, 50, 101
anti-depressants, 66, 195, 196, 200
anti-inflammatory, 82, 84, 152, 163, 181, 256
anti-nutrients, 33–34
antibiotics, 14, 72, 92, 138, 146, 155, 163
antibiotics in livestock, 143–145
antibodies, 49, 51, 67, 68, 155, 201, 287, 288
antigens, 47
anxiety, 123, 180, 182, 196, 199, 201, 202, 204, 205, 288
apoptosis, 125, 162
artificial sweetener, 121, 133, 182–184, 188, 199
autoimmune disease/ autoimmune diseases, 23–25, 26, 48, 49, 51, 67–69, 156, 286
avocado, 90, 91, 160, 164, 192

## B

back injury, 223
balance, 217–221
ballistic stretching, 226
barley, 46, 48, 51, 170, 192
bass, 93, 152
beans, 21–23, 25, 27–29, 31, 34–37, 39, 76, 101, 158, 175, 178, 292
beef, 86, 138, 139–147
beer, 109, 170
bipolar disorder, 204
birth control pills, 65–67
bison, 86, 292
black tea, 181
blood-brain barrier, 198, 201
blood glucose, 47, 51, 292

blood lipids, 87, 93, 138
blood type diet, 15
bodyweight, 141, 161, 224, 266, 273
bone density, 60
bovine growth hormone, 58, 65
brain size, 85
breast cancer, 30, 151
buckwheat, 53
butter, 74, 97, 140, 159, 177, 178, 189
B vitamins, 27, 34, 168

## C

caffeine, 179–182, 184, 199
calcium, 59, 64, 69, 82, 90, 287
cancer, 63–64, 124–127
canola oil, 5, 19, 75, 78, 85, 88, 89
carbohydrates, 35–36, 50–51, 101–114
carcinogenic, 96, 154, 156, 165
cardiac procedure, 77
cardiovascular disease, 83, 84, 91, 123, 178, 181, 216
cardiovascular health, 75, 81, 159
casomorphin, 73
catfish, 93, 152
caveman caution, 18–19
caveman moderation, 17–18
cavities, 2, 41, 42, 123, 180
celiac disease, 39, 48, 49
cellulose, 115–117
CHD, 81, 106, 172
cheese, 73–74
chicken, 14, 44, 86, 144, 146–148
chocolate, 178–179
cholesterol, 93–99
chromosomal DNA, 209
cis, 80
CLA, 82, 91
coconut, 91, 192
cod, 92, 152
coenzyme Q10, 95
coffee, 179–182
collagen, 109, 181
colon, 42–45, 106, 155
conception, 71, 258
conformity, 8, 9, 42
conjugated fatty acid, 82
conjugated linoleic acid, 82
constipation, 42–45
cooking, 184–185
corn oil, 85, 87, 90, 96, 150, 164
corn syrup, 111, 175, 176, 179
coronary heart disease, 106, 153
cortisol, 67, 132, 204, 205
cross-training, 251–252

CrossFit, 132
cytokines, 98, 200, 201

**D**

defecation, 43, 44
dental caries, 2
depression, 196, 199–207
dextrose, 111, 116
DHA, 84–86, 88, 91–93, 151, 152, 199, 200
diabetes, 24, 41, 46, 67–69, 73, 77, 92, 106, 153
digestion inhibitors, 21, 46–47
disaccharides, 115, 116–117
DNA, 11, 107–109, 135, 154, 209, 211
docosahexaenoic acid, 84–86, 88, 91–93, 151, 152, 199, 200
Dogtor J, 7, 10, 41
dynamic stretching, 225, 226, 238–243

**E**

ear infection, 3, 69, 70
eggs, 152–153, 188–189
eicosapentaenoic acid, 84–86, 91, 93, 151, 152, 190
endocrine disruptors, 29–33
endothelium, 105
EPA, 84–86, 91, 93, 151, 152, 190
epigenetic, 30, 209
epigenetics of exercise, 211–212
erectile dysfunction, 32, 106, 149
estradiol, 124, 141, 142
estrogen, 31, 32, 67, 140, 148, 150, 151
evolution, 13–15, 117–118
evolutionary self protection, 19–21
exercise, 205, 211–213, 289
extended exercise, 95, 96

**F**

farm-raised fish, 86, 92, 152, 188
fatty acid, 80, 83, 135
fertility, 20, 33, 71, 73, 92, 150, 151, 177
fiber, 42–45
fish oil, 293
flax, 87, 88, 90, 190
flexibility, 223–243
food pyramid, 157–166
free-range, 138, 143, 152, 155, 163, 179
free radicals, 84, 95, 96, 107, 108, 149
fructose, 111–113, 116, 117, 124, 132, 175, 176, 179
fruit juice, 105, 113, 137, 157, 176
frying, 82, 84, 88, 89, 91, 93, 95, 96, 164, 198

**G**

galactose, 70, 71, 116
gallstones, 124

gastrocolic reflex, 43
genetic adaptation, 56, 169
genistein, 30
ghrelin, 112, 116, 292
glucagon, 104
glucose, 50, 70, 97, 103–105, 111, 112, 116, 117, 124, 126, 129, 292
gluten, 48–51
glycation, 95, 97, 98, 103–105
glycemic index, 103, 104, 169, 191
glycemic load, 50–51, 103–106
glycerides, 79–80
glycerol, 79–81
glycogen, 16, 104, 111, 113
gout, 124
grass-fed, 91, 138, 143, 163
green tea, 181
gut bacteria, 6, 22, 31, 32, 115, 201, 202, 292, 293
gut flora, 19, 57, 177

**H**

HDL, 94–96
HDL-3, 83, 91
heart disease, 73, 74, 78, 81, 83, 85, 90, 95–97, 99, 106, 114, 153, 163, 165, 177, 180, 181, 202, 204
herring, 59, 92, 93, 188
high-glycemic, 75, 103–106, 109, 149, 150, 158, 159, 163, 168, 191
high blood pressure, 5, 77, 78, 154, 170–173
high density lipoprotein, 94
high fructose corn syrup, 112, 175, 176, 179
high intensity interval training, 246–251, 253, 259, 281
HIIT, 246–251, 253, 259, 281
hip fracture, 59, 63
honey, 17, 112, 127, 176, 177, 179, 192
hormonal disruptors, 20, 27
hydrogenated, 81, 89, 90, 159, 164, 179
hydrogenation, 81
hypertrophy, 251

**I**

ice cream, 14, 17, 64, 70, 127, 151, 191, 286
immortality switch, 125
impotence, 6, 32
infertility, 70–71
inflammation, 97, 98, 170, 180, 196
insanity, 78
insulin, 68, 72, 73, 104, 106, 107, 172, 292
insulin resistance, 47, 53, 74, 98, 105, 111, 128, 129, 131, 171–173, 292
intentionality, 18

interesterification, 81
interesterified fat, 81
intestinal bacteria, 36, 82, 154
intestinal flora, 71–73, 145
iron, 34, 45, 46, 103, 180, 260, 278
isoflavones, 31

**K**

kamut, 51
ketchup, 174, 190
ketogenic diet, 126, 127, 175
kidney stones, 124

**L**

lactase persistence, 56
lactic acid fermentation, 37
lactose, 6, 14, 15, 19, 55, 64, 70–73, 116, 159, 177, 179, 189
lactose intolerance, 56, 57
lard, 75, 78, 79, 83, 164
laxative, 7, 43, 44, 293
LDL, 94–96
LDL-B, 83, 91
lectin/lectins, 22–25, 47–48
legumes, 27–37
leptin resistance, 47, 128, 129, 131, 132, 292
linseed, 83, 88
liquor, 109, 178
liver, 43, 93–95, 97, 104, 109, 111, 112, 116, 124, 132, 153, 170, 180
low density lipoprotein, 94–96
lupus, 49

**M**

mackerel, 92, 152, 155, 188, 190
macular degeneration, 106, 114, 165, 182, 183
maple syrup, 130, 175
maximum effort, 247–248
mayonnaise, 174–175, 188, 190
mercury, 8, 86, 92, 152, 188
metabolic disorder, 13, 123, 127
metabolic pathway, 84, 95, 175
microbiological safety, 145–148, 156
micronutrients, 173, 193
milk, 55–74, 177–178
millet, 51
mitochondria, 107
mitochondrial DNA, 108, 109
monosaccharides, 116–117
monounsaturated, 78–80, 83, 86, 87, 90, 138, 139
mucus, 23, 44, 47, 70, 155
multiple sclerosis, 68, 69, 73, 92, 177
muscle, 16, 104, 111, 122, 164, 168, 211, 223–227, 255–257

mustard, 174, 190, 206
myelin, 69, 93
my plate, 45, 157

**N**

negative reps, 255–256, 260, 270, 271
neurological recruitment, 257
neurotransmitters, 120, 129, 133, 195, 196, 292
NHEL, 141, 142
nightshade, 286–288
nitrites, 152–156, 163, 165, 170, 188
nitrosamines, 154–156, 165
NOEL, 143
no hormonal effect level, 141, 142
no observable effect level, 143
NSAID, 170

**O**

obesity, 32, 47, 50, 51, 57, 75, 125, 171, 202, 204, 206, 210
oleic acid, 83
oligosaccharide, 36, 37
olive oil, 78, 83, 87, 88, 90, 91, 93, 138, 160, 164, 174, 175, 187, 190
omega-3, 137–139
omega-6, 137–139
organic, 50, 58, 122, 138, 143, 155, 163, 179, 187–190
osteoporosis, 58–60
ovarian cancer, 63–64, 73, 74
ovulatory infertility, 71, 74, 106
oxidation, 83, 95, 98, 103
oxidative stress, 82, 84, 96
oxidize, 80, 82, 88, 96, 97, 112, 153

**P**

palm, 239, 268, 273
Parkinson's disease, 69
pasteurized, 58, 60–63
peanuts, 23, 69, 102, 159, 191
peas, 31, 158
phytase, 22, 37
phytic acid, 21–23, 33, 34, 37, 45, 52, 53
phyto-estrogens, 30–33
phytohaemagglutinin, 21, 27–28, 35
polysaccharides, 115
polyunsaturated, 78–84, 86–91, 93, 95, 96, 98, 137–139, 149, 159, 174, 200
pork, 138–139, 143, 144, 146, 164
potassium chloride, 193
potato/potatoes, 22, 102, 111, 113, 115, 140, 168, 287
power, 245–284
probiotic, 37, 293
progesterone, 140–142
prolamines, 51

proprioception, 217–221
prostate cancer, 30, 63, 64, 150, 151, 165, 180
protease inhibitors, 35
protein, 23, 35, 68–70, 97, 135, 136, 150, 154, 156–163
psoriasis, 49
psychosomatic, 57

**Q**
quinoa, 53

**R**
raw milk, 60–63
rheumatoid arthritis, 24, 49
risk factors, 24, 25, 92, 182, 183, 216
Ritalin, 196
root vegetables, 113, 114, 147
rust, 103
rye, 45, 48, 51, 192

**S**
sabotage, 290–291
salad, 174–175
salmon, 59, 92, 131, 139, 152, 155, 162, 163, 188, 190
salt, 170–173
saponins, 28
sardines, 59, 87, 92, 138, 139, 152, 155, 188, 190
satiety, 47, 114, 116, 128, 161, 169
saturated fat, 73, 78, 79, 82, 83, 87, 91, 114, 138, 153, 159
seafood, 151–152, 188
sea salt, 173, 191
sitting, 214–217
sleep, 204–205
sleep apnea, 132
solvents, 87–90
soreness, 256–257
sorghum, 39, 51
sourdough, 39, 52
soy, 27, 175
soybean oil, 87, 152, 164, 174, 179, 188, 200
soy sauce, 175
spelt, 51, 192
sperm, 71
sperm count, 31, 32, 106
spices, 187, 192, 291
starchy roots, 168
static stretches, 224–227, 273, 279
statin, 5, 6, 43, 44, 95, 198, 293
steak sauce, 174
stimulants, 44, 180, 196
strength, 245–284
stress, 64–67, 82, 84, 94, 96, 98
stroke, 74, 106, 153, 165, 181
sucrose, 111, 117, 124, 199, 202

sugar, 115–116, 121–130,
sugar addiction, 127–130
suicide/suicides, 125, 162, 196, 200, 202
sunflower oil, 83, 87, 190
sunshine, 69, 93, 206–207, 294
supplements, 293–294

**T**
table sugar, 111–113, 117, 124, 175, 176
tallow, 83, 164
tapioca, 16, 167, 168
tea, 179–182
telomeres, 125
testosterone, 32, 67, 140–142, 148, 149, 205
tooth decay, 41–42
trace minerals, 89, 173
tranquilizers, 66, 195, 196
trans fat/trans fats, 81, 84, 89, 90, 182, 196, 197
triglycerides, 79–81, 96, 112, 153, 163
trout, 93, 152
tuberculosis, 61
tuna, 86, 92, 139, 152, 156, 164, 188
TV, 55, 113, 132, 191, 196, 202–204, 207, 213
type I diabetes, 67–69, 92, 177
type II diabetes, 74, 180

**U**
ulcers, 8, 9, 23
unsaturated, 80, 82, 83, 90, 139, 159

**V**
vaccenic acid, 80
veganism, 136, 137
vegetarian, 5, 18
venison, 86
vinegar, 169
vitamin C, 95, 103, 154, 157, 165
vitamin D, 4, 69, 74, 93, 206, 207, 293, 294

**W**
walking, 214–217
walnut, 87
warm-up, 224–226, 23/
wheat, 5, 7, 39, 45–48, 94, 155, 175, 189, 191, 192
whitefish, 93
white rice, 52, 113, 114, 168
white tea, 181
wild seafood, 92, 152
wine, 90, 109, 170
Worcestershire sauce, 175
wrinkles, 65, 108–110

**Y**
yogurt, 71–73
yolk, 93